Central

one week loan

Please return on or before the last
date stamped below.
Charges are made for late return.

IS 238/0199

INFORMATION SERVICES PO BOX 430, CARDIFF CF1 3XT

PRACTICAL ASPECTS OF OPHTHALMIC OPTICS

Fourth Edition

Margaret Dowaliby, O.D.
Professor, Professional Studies (Ret.)
Southern California College of Optometry

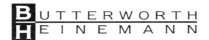

Boston Oxford Auckland Johannesburg Melbourne New Delhi

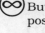 Recognizing the importance of preserving what has been written, Butterworth–Heinemann prints its books on acid-free paper whenever possible.

 Butterworth–Heinemann supports the efforts of American Forests and the Global ReLeaf program in its campaign for the betterment of trees, forests, and our environment.

Library of Congress Cataloging-in-Publication Data
Dowaliby, Margaret.
    Practical aspects of ophthalmic optics / Margaret Dowaliby.—4th ed.
        p. cm.
    Includes index.
    ISBN 0-7506-7189-0 (alk. paper)
    1. Optometry. 2. Physiological optics. I. Title.

    RE951 .D68 2000
    617.7'5—dc21   00-060890

British Library Cataloguing-in-Publication Data
A catalogue record for this book is available from the British Library.

The publisher offers special discounts on bulk orders of this book. For information, please contact:

Manager of Special Sales
Butterworth–Heinemann
225 Wildwood Avenue
Woburn, MA 01801-2041
Tel: 781-904-2500
Fax: 781-904-2620

For information on all Butterworth–Heinemann publications available, contact our World Wide Web home page at: http://www.bh.com
10 9 8 7 6 5 4 3 2 1
Printed in the United States of America

To my mother, Hend

Whose love I remember more and more
as the years go by

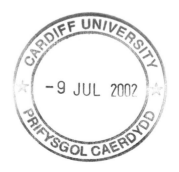

CONTENTS

When contemplating a new preface for this update of *Practical Aspects of Ophthalmic Optics*, I was surprised upon reading and rereading the preface for the previous edition that I could not improve upon it. Advances in the field of ophthalmic optics are even greater, startling in fact, because there are so many lens and frame additions (and some deletions). They appear with such regularity that the eyecare professional needs to constantly pursue the new literature distributed by the optical manufacturers.

However, the basics remain the same, and this book reflects what is necessary for eyecare professionals to make the right choice for their patients. The material is presented in an easy-to-understand format that I believe is invaluable to both student and practitioner.

PREFACE

Eyecare as it is known today, with all the possibilities involved in providing visual efficiency, is to a large degree the result of tremendous strides made in the field of ophthalmic optics. Advances in the design of conventional ophthalmic lenses have resulted in an optical efficiency that until recently was within the realm of improbability. Progress in the area of unusual lens design has made it possible for many patients to enjoy visual corrections that previously presented optical and cosmetic problems.

By classic definition, ophthalmic optics is that aspect of geometric and physical optics dealing with the application of lenses to the human eye. The contemporary field of ophthalmic optics involves itself with designs of lenses mounted in frames (eyewear), lenses worn within the conjunctival sac (contact lenses), and lenses worn as magnifying units (low-vision aids). Each of these types of visual correction has undergone dramatic improvement in the past decade. To explain the advancements fully, books need to be devoted to each area. This volume concerns itself solely with lenses mounted into conventional eyeframes. It is highly practical in nature and involves itself with the optics of today's wide range of lens designs. Some lenses are simple, some complex, but each in its own way serves as the best possible visual aid for the care of a specific patient.

This area is of primary concern to most practitioners because the majority of patients seeking visual care are aided by a correction in the form of conventional eyewear. This book discusses the changes in single-vision lenses, the constantly expanding field of multifocal prescribing, the advances in the field of safety eyewear, the complexities in today's world of absorptive lenses, and the growing expansion of aids that make lenses optically superior as well as cosmetically pleasing.

This book's goals are to give the practitioner the opportunity to reevaluate the availability of optical products that best serve the patient and to acquaint the student with the practical aspects involved in the field of ophthalmic optics. It needs to be kept in mind that availability of product has become so great that while optic principles will always stay the same, application to specific lens/frame designs may change.

In preparing this update of *Practical Aspects of Ophthalmic Optics* I was struck by how often there was more "hype" about product than actual specifics. Yet the specifics must be understood if patients are to receive maximum benefits. Studying this text, studying the released literature accompanying products, applying the principles discussed in the text, and keeping abreast of changes through the local optical laboratory will result in the eyecare professional's ability to recommend the most suitable lens/frame designs for patients' enjoyment of their eyewear.

ACKNOWLEDGMENTS

I am deeply grateful to those in the optical field who helped me verify certain sections of this update of *Practical Aspects of Ophthalmic Optics*.

I am especially thankful to Joseph Bruneni, faculty member, Southern California College of Optometry, whose extensive writings in the field of ophthalmic optics proved invaluable in compiling the material for this book.

There were also others whose help in their respective specialties proved most important: David Hernendez, Younger Optics; Russell Evans and Frank Yaeger, also of Younger Optics; Grady Culbreth, Carl Zeiss Optical, Inc.; Darryl Meister, Sola Optical USA, and Dr. Rod Tehran, Varilux.

Special mention to Sue Klein of Vision-Ease Lens who always extended her expertise in the area of lens designs; and to Michael Randy Dowaliby, optician, Beverly Hills, CA. Particular thanks to Cindy Berman who helped prepare the manuscript for publication.

Chapter 1

CHARACTERISTICS OF LENSES

INTRODUCTION

An ophthalmic lens is a transparent medium bound by two polished surfaces, either plane or curved, that act as an optical system. Two substances are used in the production of lenses: glass, until recently the most widely prescribed, and plastic, which is recommended with increasing frequency.

Modern ophthalmic lenses are prescribed for many reasons. Their primary use is the correction of refractive errors. They also may aid in correcting faulty binocular vision. They may act as protection against foreign objects. Some designs serve as absorptive lenses to filter those portions of the spectrum that prove uncomfortable or harmful to the patient.

Refractive errors result when light rays entering the eye do not focus on the retina. Basically three conditions exist: hyperopia, or far-sightedness; myopia, or near-sightedness; and astigmatism.

In cases of hyperopia, light rays entering the eye focus behind the retina and must be converged to provide clear, comfortable vision. This is accomplished by prescribing plus (convex) lenses, which exhibit the following characteristics:

1. A plus lens converges parallel light. If the light is converging as it passes through the lens, the convergence

is increased; if it is diverging, either it diverges less or it may converge, depending upon the power of the lens.

2.   Parallel rays of light passing through a plus lens will focus at a specific distance, depending upon the power of the lens.

3.   The center thickness of a plus lens is greater than its edge thickness.

4.   When the observer views an object through a plus lens, the image is magnified.

5.   When a plus lens is held before the eye so that the secondary focal point falls behind the retina, a movement of the lens results in an opposite motion of objects viewed through the lens. This movement is technically referred to as "against motion."

6.   The effective power of a plus lens increases as it is moved away from the eye.

In cases of myopia, light rays entering the eye focus in front of the retina. To correct this anomaly, minus lenses are prescribed. These concave lenses demonstrate the following characteristics:

1.   Minus lenses diverge parallel light. If the light is diverging as it passes through the lens, the divergence increases; if converging, it will converge less or diverge, depending upon the power of the lens.

2.   Light incident upon a minus lens will not come to a point focus.

3.   Objects viewed through a concave lens are minified.

4.   The edge thickness of a minus lens is greater than its center thickness.

5.   When a minus lens is held before the eye, the object viewed moves in the same direction as the movement of the lens. This technically is referred to as *with motion.*

6.   The effective power of a minus lens decreases as it is moved away from the eye.

In cases of astigmatism, light rays entering the eye are not focused at a single point but instead focus as two line images at right angles to each other. This anomaly, known as *regular astigmatism*, requires a correcting lens with power that gradually increases from a minimum in one meridian to the maximum amount in the meridian 90° away. These are known as the *principal meridians of the lens* and coincide with the major meridians of the eye. The correcting lenses for regular astigmatism are known as *cylinders* and have the following characteristics:

1. A conventional cylindrical lens has one toric surface (a surface having meridians of least and greatest curvature located at right angles to each other).

2. The meridian of least power is known as the axis; the meridian of maximum power is 90° away. In this 90° span there is a gradual increase in the power of the cylinder, the amount dependent on the angle subtended from the axis.

3. When a line object is viewed through a cylinder so that the axis or the meridian of greatest power coincides with that line, rotation of the lens produces a "break" in its continuity. If the motion of the line is opposite to the movement of the lens, the meridian involved is the plus cylinder axis or the meridian of least plus power. Conversely, if the movement is in the same direction, the meridian is the minus cylinder axis or the meridian of most plus power.

Note: There is another type of astigmatism, relatively rare and known as *irregular astigmatism*, in which the two principal meridians of the eye are not 90° apart. Cylindrical lenses cannot fully correct this anomaly.

DESIGNATION OF LENS POWER

The basic unit of power for lenses is the diopter, usually abbreviated as D. By definition, the number of diopters of power is equal to the reciprocal of the focal length of the lens in meters. Therefore, the formula for dioptric power is stated as follows:

$$1/\text{focal length (meters)} = \text{diopters}$$

Example:

If the focal length of a lens is 1 meter, then $1/1\text{m} = 1.00\text{D}$. If the focal length is 40 centimeters, then $1/.4\text{m} = 2.50\text{D}$.

Conversely, the focal length of a lens can be found by taking the reciprocal of its dioptric power:

$$1/\text{diopters} = \text{focal length (meters)}$$

Example:

If the lens power is +3.00 diopters, then 1/3.00D = 33.3 centimeters.

If the lens power is +0.25 diopters, then 1/0.25D = 4 meters.

Note: Focal length is measured from the *back* surface of the lens to the point of focus. This interval is known as the *vertex focal distance*. Therefore, the stated dioptric power of an ophthalmic lens is actually the vertex power.

POWER OF LENSES

Ophthalmic lenses are manufactured in 1/8D intervals. This difference has been found to be the smallest increment discernible to the patient, although quarter-diopter steps present a degree of accuracy sufficient in most cases. Thus, the available dioptric range of ophthalmic lenses includes plano (no power, but possessing the quality optical characteristics), +0.12D, +0.25D, +0.37D, +0.50D, +0.62D, +0.75D, +0.87D, +1.00D, +1.12D, +1.25D, etc.; and −0.12D, −0.25D, −0.37D, etc.

OTHER LENS CLASSIFICATIONS

Spherical Lenses

Ophthalmic lenses are also classified as spheres, plano-cylinders, and sphero-cylinders (combination of sphere and cylinder).

Spherical lenses are designated as such because their curved surfaces are similar to sections of a sphere. The same refractive power is found in all meridians and, depending on the prescription, the lens may converge light (plus or convex lenses), diverge light (minus or concave lenses), or leave parallel rays unaltered (plano lenses).

Plano-cylindrical Lenses

A plano-cylindrical lens has one meridian that contains no power; it is known as the axis and is the reference meridian of all cylindrical lenses. Ninety degrees away from the axis is the toroidal meridian of maximum power. In the other meridians, the cylinder power varies between the axis and the meridian of maximum curvature according to the following formula:

$$F´ = F_{\text{total cylinder}} \times \sin^2 \Theta$$

$F´$ = cylinder power of any given meridian

$F_{\text{total cylinder}}$ = total power of the cylinder

Θ = angle between the axis and the meridian in question

The powers of five meridians in a plano-cylindrical lens are easily calculated. When these are known, it is possible to estimate rather accurately the power in any other meridian. Applying the formula $F´= F (\sin^2 \Theta)$, the power 30° away from the axis is equal to $^1/_4$ of the total power of the cylinder; 45° away, $^1/_2$ the power; and 60° away, $^3/_4$ of the total cylindrical power.

The simplicity of computing the powers in the meridians mentioned is illustrated by the following examples:

PROBLEM:

Given a −2.00 × 30° lens, find the power in the following meridians: (a) 180°, (b) 30°, (c) 60°, (d) 90°, (e) 120°.

SOLUTION:

$F´ = F (\sin^2 \Theta)$
(a) $F´ = (-2.00) (\sin^2 30°) = (-2.00) (0.25) = -0.50D$
(b) $F´ = (-2.00) (\sin^2 \Theta) = (-2.00) (0.00) = -0.00D$
(c) $F´ = (-2.00) (\sin^2 30°) = (-2.00) (0.25) = -0.50D$
(d) $F´ = (-2.00) (\sin^2 60°) = (-2.00) (0.75) = -1.50D$
(e) $F´ = (-2.00) (\sin^2 90°) = (-2.00) (1.00) = -2.00D$

PROBLEM:

Given a plano +1.00 cylindrical lens with axis 90°, compute the powers in the following meridians: (a) 90°, (b) 60°, (c) 45°, (d) 30°, (e) 180°.

SOLUTION:

(a) Plano at 90° (no power at axis)
(b) +0.25D at 60° ($^1/_4$ of +1.00D, 30° from axis)
(c) +0.50D at 45° ($^1/_2$ of +1.00D, 45° from axis)

(d) +0.75D at 30° ($^3/_4$ of +1.00D, 60° from axis)
(e) +1.00D at 180° (total power 90° from axis)

If accurate power in meridians not 30°, 45°, 60°, or 90° from the axis is desired, it is necessary to utilize the formula given: $F' = F (\sin^2 \Theta)$.

PROBLEM:

Given a $-1.00 \times 180°$ lens, find the power in the following meridians: (a) 180°, (b) 5°, (c) 15°, (d) 25°, (e) 30°, (f) 40°, (g) 45°, (h) 55°, (i) 60°, (j)70°, (k) 80°, (l) 90°.

SOLUTION:

$F' = F (\sin^2\Theta)$
(a) $F' = (-1.00) (\sin^2 0°) = (-1.00) (0.00) = 0.00D$
(b) $F' = (-1.00) (\sin^2 5°) = (-1.00) (0.01) = -0.01D$
(c) $F' = (-1.00) (\sin^2 15°) = (-1.00) (0.07) = -0.07D$
(d) $F' = (-1.00) (\sin^2 25°) = (-1.00) (0.18) = -0.18D$
(e) $F' = (-1.00) (\sin^2 30°) = (-1.00) (0.25) = -0.25D$
(f) $F' = (-1.00) (\sin^2 40°) = (-1.00) (0.41) = -0.41D$
(g) $F' = (-1.00) (\sin^2 45°) = (-1.00) (0.50) = -0.50D$
(h) $F' = (-1.00) (\sin^2 55°) = (-1.00) (0.67) = -0.67D$
(i) $F' = (-1.00) (\sin^2 60°) = (-1.00) (0.75) = -0.75D$
(j) $F' = (-1.00) (\sin^2 70°) = (-1.00) (0.88) = -0.88D$
(k) $F' = (-1.00) (\sin^2 80°) = (-1.00) (0.97) = -0.97D$
(l) $F' = (-1.00) (\sin^2 90°) = (-1.00) (1.00) = -1.00D$

Sphero-cylindrical Lenses

Sphero-cylindrical lenses have a spherical component that is found throughout the lens. To determine the total power in a particular meridian, the cylinder is computed in the manner previously discussed and added to the sphere.

PROBLEM:

Given a $+3.00 + 1.00 \times 90°$ lens, find the power in the following meridians: (a) 90°, (b) 60°, (c) 45°, (d) 30°, (e) 180°.

SOLUTION:

$F' = F_{sphere} + F_{cylinder} (\sin^2 \Theta)$
(a) $F' = +3.00 + (+1.00) (\sin^2 0°) = +3.00D$
(b) $F' = +3.00 + (+1.00) (\sin^2 30°) = +3.25D$

(c) $F´ = +3.00 + (+1.00) (\sin^2 45°) = +3.50D$
(d) $F´ = +3.00 + (+1.00) (\sin^2 60°) = +3.75D$
(e) $F´ = +3.00 + (+1.00) (\sin^2 90°) = +4.00D$

PROBLEM:

Given a $+3.00 - 3.00 \times 60°$ lens, find the power in the following meridians: (a) 60°, (b) 90°, (c) 105°, (d) 120°, (e) 150°.

SOLUTION:

$F´ = F_{sphere} (\sin^2 \Theta)$
(a) $F´ = +3.00 + (-3.00) (\sin^2 0°)$
$= +3.00 + (-3.00) (0.00) = +3.00D$
(b) $F´ = +3.00 + (-3.00) (\sin^2 30°)$
$= +3.00 + (-3.00) (0.25) = +2.25D$
(c) $F´ = +3.00 + (-3.00) (\sin^2 45°)$
$= +3.00 + (-3.00) (0.50) = +1.50D$
(d) $F´ = +3.00 + (-3.00) (\sin^2 60°)$
$= +3.00 + (-3.00) (0.75) = +.75D$
(e) $F´ = +3.00 + (-3.00) (\sin^2 90°)$
$= +3.00 + (-3.00) (1.00) = +0.00D$

PROBLEM:

Given a $-4.00 - 1.00 \times 180°$ lens, find the power in the following meridians: (a) 180°, (b) 30°, (c) 45°, (d) 60°, (e) 90°.

SOLUTION:

$F´ = F_{sphere} + F_{cylinder} (\sin^2 \Theta)$
(a) $F´ = -4.00 + (-1.00) (\sin^2 0°)$
$= -4.00 + (-0.00) = -4.00D$
(b) $F´ = -4.00 + (-1.00) (\sin^2 30°)$
$= -4.00 + (-1.00) (0.25) = -4.25D$
(c) $F´ = -4.00 + (-1.00) (\sin^2 45°)$
$= -4.00 + (-1.00) (0.50) = -4.50D$
(d) $F´ = -4.00 + (-1.00) (\sin^2 60°)$
$= -4.00 + (-1.00) (0.75) = -4.75D$
(e) $F´ = -4.00 + (-1.00) (\sin^2 90°)$
$= -4.00 + (-1.00) (1.00) = -5.00D$

The cylinder power of a plano-cylinder or sphero-cylinder lens can be ground on either the convex or concave surface, but manufacturers, with rare exception, have phased out plus-cylinder lenses because minus designs keep meridional magnification at a minimum.

In cases of high-power cylinder prescriptions, minus cylinders offer a definite cosmetic advantage. Since the changes in curvature to accommodate the cylinder are on the back surface, the thickness difference is not as apparent when the glasses are worn.

The cylinder form of a multifocal lens is predetermined by the design, and the cylindrical surface is always on the side opposite the segment.

WRITING THE PRESCRIPTION

An ophthalmic prescription is correctly written to two decimal places. If less than 1 diopter of power is involved, it is customary in some areas to precede the decimal point with a zero. For example, a quarter-diopter of power could be written as 0.25D.

The spherical power is first noted, sometimes followed by the diopters of sphere (D.S.). The next quotation is the cylinder, which may be affixed to the diopters of cylinder (D.C.). The axis is preceded by a multiplication sign and is sometimes followed by a degree sign. For example:

$$+2.00 \text{ D.S.} - 3.00 \text{ D.C.} \times 90°$$

However, for simplicity, when writing the prescription, it is customary to omit *D.S.*, *D.C.*, and the degree sign. The prescription then reads as follows:

$$+2.00 - 3.00 \times 90$$

It is usually best to eliminate the degree sign because it can be mistaken for a zero. For example, note that the prescription $+1.00 + 4.25 \times 10°$ could be mistaken for $+1.00 + 4.25 \times 100$ if the degree sign were not in correct proportion to the other numbers.

TRANSPOSITION

Practitioners usually write the prescription in the same cylinder form they used when examining the patient with the refractor. However, because most laboratories now use minus-cylinder, single-vision lenses and multifocals have a predetermined cylinder form, it may be necessary to convert the written prescription from plus to minus cylinders (or vice versa) without actually changing the lens power. This conversion is known as "transposition." Plano-cylinder and sphero-cylinder lenses are transposed by the following method:

1. Add the powers of the sphere and cylinder algebraically. If the lens is a plano-cylinder, the sphere power is noted as zero.
2. Change the sign of the cylinder retaining the same amount of cylinder.
3. Add or subtract 90°, whichever leaves the axis 180° or less.

Sometimes the principal meridians of the eye are refracted with spherical lenses. This may be necessary when trial lens examinations are performed (i.e., for small children or "home refractions" for invalids). The prescription may originally be recorded as two crossed cylinders with the axes positioned 90° apart. For example, if +1.00D neutralizes the horizontal meridian of the eye and +3.00D neutralizes the vertical, the result is +1.00 × 90° ⊃ + 3.00 × 180°. The crossed-cylinder prescription is then transposed into sphero-cylinder form.

The following is the procedure for transposing into plus cylinder form:

1. Transpose the lowest plus cylinder so that both axes are the same:

    $$+1.00 \times 90° \text{ becomes } +1.00 - 1.00 \times 180°$$

2. Algebraically add the transposed +1.00 − 1.00 × 180° to the remaining plano-cylinder retaining the same axis:

$$
\begin{array}{r}
-1.00 - 1.00 \times 180° \\
+3.00 \times 180° \\
\hline
+1.00 + 2.00 \times 180°
\end{array}
$$

To transpose into minus cylinder form, transpose +1.00 + 2.00 × 180° into +3.00 − 2.00 × 90° by the procedure outlined earlier in this chapter.

A sphero-cylinder prescription can be changed to cross-cylinders 90° to each other. The following problem shows the procedure.

PROBLEM:

Transpose $+1.00 + 2.00 \times 180°$ into cross-cylinder form.

PROCEDURE:

1.   Record the sphere as a cylinder, axis 90° away from the original:

$$+1.00 \times 90°$$

2.   Add the original sphere and cylinder algebraically and record as a cylinder at the original axis:

$$+3.00 \times 180°$$

3.   Combine the answers for (1) and (2).

SOLUTION:

$$+1.00 \times 90° \supset \; +3.00 \times 180°$$

COMBINING TWO CROSS CYLINDERS THAT ARE NOT 90° APART

It is extremely rare, but possible, for a prescription to be written with the cylinders not positioned 90° apart. The prescription needs to be rewritten in sphero-cylinder form before the lens can be manufactured. There are two methods by which this can be accomplished. One is a graphic procedure; the other is a formula method. Two examples of each are given.

PROBLEM I:

What is the plus sphero-cylinder equivalent of the following prescription?

$$+3.00 \times 55° \supset \; +1.00 \times 50°$$

GRAPHIC PROCEDURE:

1. The cylinder powers are graphed along an A line and a B line. The A cylinder has the axis closest to the numerical value zero.

$$A \text{ cylinder} = +1.00 \times 50°$$

$$B \text{ cylinder} = +3.00 \times 55°$$

2. Cylinder A is plotted on the base line. Cylinder B is plotted 2α degrees away. α is the difference between the two axes (55° – 50°); in this case $\alpha = 5°$.

$$2\alpha = 10°$$

3. Graph cylinder A and cylinder B, and complete the parallelogram by drawing a dotted line from the point of origin to the opposite extremity of the parallelogram (Figure 1.1).

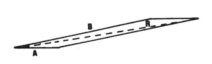

FIGURE 1.1

4. The dotted line R represents the resultant cylinder, and R measured = +4.00D.

5. The new sphere (S) is determined with the formula

$$S = \frac{A_{cyl} + B_{cyl} - R_{cyl}}{2}$$

$$S = \frac{+1.00 + 3.00 - 4.00}{2}$$

$$= 0.00D$$

6. The new axis is the axis of cylinder A plus γ. The angle between A and R is 2γ (measured 8°).

$$\gamma = 4°$$

The new axis is 54° (50° + 4°).

GRAPHIC SOLUTION TO PROBLEM I:

Plus sphero-cylinder equivalent = plano +4.00 × 54°

FORMULA PROCEDURE:

For solving a cross-cylinder problem by the formula method, the following trigonometric functions need to be considered:
In the first quadrant all functions are positive.
In the second quadrant the sine only is positive.
In the third quadrant the tangent only is positive.
In the fourth quadrants the cosine only is positive.

1. The formula for the resultant cylinder is

$$R_{cyl} = \sqrt{A^2 + B^2 + 2AB \cos 2\alpha}$$

If 2α is less than 90°, the formula stays as above. If 2α is exactly 90°, the term $2AB \cos 2\alpha$ drops and the formula reads $R_{cyl} = \sqrt{A^2 + B^2}$ (because cos 90° = 0). If 2α is more than 90°, the cosine term becomes negative (cosine is negative in the second quadrant). The formula now reads:

$$R_{cyl} = \sqrt{A^2 + B^2 - 2AB \cos 2\alpha}$$

In this problem the first formula applies because 2α is less than 90°.

$$R_{cyl} = \sqrt{A^2 + B^2 + 2AB \cos 2\alpha}$$
$$= \sqrt{1^2 + 3^2 + 2(1)(3)\cos 10°}$$
$$= \sqrt{15.91}$$
$$= 3.99D$$

2. The sphere is determined with the formula

$$S = \frac{A_{cyl} + B_{cyl} - R_{cyl}}{2}$$

$$= \frac{+1.00 + 3.00 - 3.99}{2}$$

$$= +0.005D$$

3. The new axis is determined with the formula A axis + γ, and γ is found with the formula

$$\frac{\sin 2\gamma}{B_{cyl}} = \frac{\sin 2\alpha}{R_{cyl}}$$

$$\frac{\sin 2\gamma}{+3.00} = \frac{\sin 10°}{+3.99}$$

$$\sin 2\gamma = \frac{+3.00(0.17365)}{+3.99}$$

$$2\gamma = 8°$$

$$\gamma = 4°$$

4. The axis of A + γ = 50° + 4° = 54°.

FORMULA SOLUTION TO PROBLEM I:

Plus-cylinder form prescription = +0.005 + 3.99 × 54°

PROBLEM II:

Change the following prescription into plus sphero-cylinder form.

$$+3.00 \times 60° \supset -4.00 \times 25°$$

GRAPHIC PROCEDURE:

1. Transpose both cylinders to plus cylinder form. Note: Before graphing, cylinders need to be the same sign. Transposed, the formula reads:

$$+3.00 \times 60° \supset -4.00 + 4.00 \times 115°$$

2.   The two cylinders are +3.00 × 60° $\supset$ + 4.00 × 115°. Cylinder A = +3.00D (numerical value closest to zero). Cylinder B = +4.00D.

$$\alpha = 115° - 60° = 55°$$
$$2\alpha = 110°$$

3.   Graph cylinder A and cylinder B and complete the parallelogram (Figure 1.2).

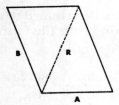

FIGURE 1.2

4.   The resultant cylinder R measures +4.10D.
5.   Determine the new sphere:

$$S = \frac{A_{cyl} + B_{cyl} - R_{cyl}}{2} + \text{original sphere (after transposition)}$$

$$= \frac{+3.00 + 4.00 - 4.10}{2} + (-4.00)$$

$$= 2.55D$$

6.   The new axis is equal to A axis + γ.

$$2\gamma = 66°$$
$$\gamma = 33°$$

The new axis is equal to 60° + 33° = 93°.

GRAPHIC SOLUTION TO PROBLEM II:

Plus cylinder prescription = −2.55 + 4.10 × 93°

FORMULA PROCEDURE:

1.   Transpose so that both cylinders are in plus-cylinder form, +3.00 × 60° $\supset$ − 4.00 + 4.00 × 115°.

2.   Cylinder A = +3.00 × 60° (numerical value of axis closest to zero). Cylinder B = +4.00 × 115°.

$$\alpha = 115° - 60° = 55°$$
$$2\alpha = 110°$$

3.   The formula for the new cylinder is

$$R_{cyl} = \sqrt{A^2 + B^2 + 2AB \cos 2\alpha}$$

$$R_{cyl} = \sqrt{3^2 + 4^2 + 2(3)(4)\cos 110°}$$

$$= \sqrt{16.9}$$

$$= +4.11D$$

4.   The new sphere is determined by

$$S = \frac{A_{cyl} + B_{cyl} - R_{cyl}}{2} + \text{original sphere}$$

$$S = \frac{+3.00 + 4.00 - 4.11}{2} + (-4.00)$$

$$= 2.56D$$

5.   Determine the new axis with the formula A axis + γ, where γ is calculated with the formula

$$\frac{\sin 2\gamma}{B_{cyl}} = \frac{\sin 2\alpha}{R_{cyl}}$$

$$\frac{\sin 2\gamma}{+4.00} = \frac{\sin 110°}{+4.11}$$

$$2\gamma = 66°$$

$$\gamma = 33°$$

Therefore, the new axis is 60° + 33° = 93°.

FORMULA SOLUTION TO PROBLEM II:

Plus cylinder prescription = −2.56 + 4.11 × 93°

OPTICAL CROSS

An optical cross is a simple cross diagram indicating the powers in the various lens meridians. Intersecting lines 90° apart representing the axis and the meridian of maximum power are always included; other lines may be used to represent meridians of special interest.

Example:

Prescriptions usually are placed on an optical cross to determine quickly the power in a particular meridian (Figures 1.3 and 1.4).

Prescriptions are placed on an optical cross by the following method:

1.   The spherical correction is noted in the principal meridians although it is understood to encompass the entire lens.
2.   The cylindrical correction is noted 90° away from the axis.
3.   The sphere and the cylinder are added algebraically in the meridian involved.

Example:

Note: It is customary to mark the powers in the upper quadrants of the cross (Figures 1.5 and 1.6), although it is understood that the entire meridian in question is involved.

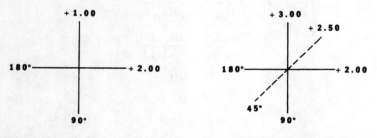

FIGURE 1.3   *+1.00 + 1.00 × 90°*   FIGURE 1.4   *+3.00 − 1.00 × 90°*

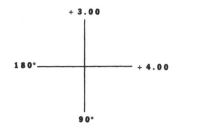

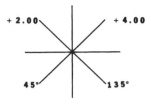

FIGURE 1.5   *+3.00 + 1.00 × 90°*   FIGURE 1.6   *+4.00 − 2.00 × 45°*

A prescription can be written three ways:

1. In plus-cylinder form
2. In minus-cylinder form
3. In cross-cylinder form

The following powers are noted on an optical cross (Figure 1.7).

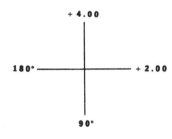

FIGURE 1.7

PROBLEM:

Write the prescription on this cross (Figure 1.7) in (a) plus-cylinder form, (b) minus-cylinder form, (c) cross-cylinder form.

SOLUTION:

$+2.00 + 2.00 × 180°$
$+4.00 − 2.00 × 90°$
$+2.00 × 90° \supset + 4.00 × 180°$

PROBLEM:

The following powers are noted on an optical cross (Figure 1.8). Write the prescription in the following three forms: (a) plus cylinder, (b) minus cylinder, (c) cross cylinder.

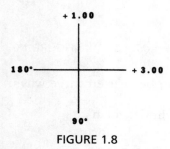

FIGURE 1.8

SOLUTION:

+1.00 + 2.00 × 90°
+3.00 − 2.00 × 180°
+3.00 × 90° ⊃ + 1.00 × 180°

POSITIONING THE CYLINDER

Cylinder meridians are designated from 0° to 180°. Viewed from the front surface (looking at the patient), meridians are noted counterclockwise (Figures 1.9 and 1.10) beginning with 0° at the patient's left and increasing to 180°.

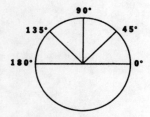

FIGURE 1.9   *Right Lens*

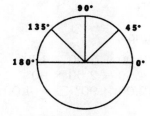

FIGURE 1.10   *Left Lens*

BASE CURVES OF SPHERICAL LENSES

Ophthalmic lenses can be grouped according to base curves. When spherical lenses are involved, the base curve is the power of one surface common to a specific lens series. With toric lenses, it is the weakest curve on the cylindrical surface. With multifocals, the base curve is the spherical curve on the segment side. The reference surface in each instance usually guarantees a standardization that manufacturers accept as a basis for the design of lenses. However, when ordering, it is best to specify the curve on the spherical side of the lens. The base curve will identify a spherical single-vision lens with one of the five conventional lens forms.

1. Plano-convex or Plano-concave

The base curve of these lenses is a plane surface with the total lens power ground on the opposite side (Figures 1.11 and 1.12). Since the flattest curve of a lens is the ocular surface, the plano-convex lens has the total power ground on the nonocular side; the plano-concave lens has the total power on the ocular surface. Use of this form is limited to high-power prescriptions, although plano-convex and plano-concave lenses are sometimes found in older trial lens sets.

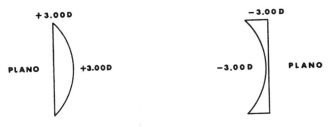

FIGURE 1.11   *Plano-convex*   FIGURE 1.12   *Plano-concave*

2. Biconvex and Biconcave

The biconvex lens features two convex surfaces usually of equal curvature (Figures 1.13 and 1.14). Similarly, the biconcave design has both surfaces usually of equal minus power. It is rare to have a biconvex or biconcave lens with different curvatures, but when it does occur, either surface may be considered the base curve. This lens form is rarely manufactured, except in trial lens sets and some low-vision aids.

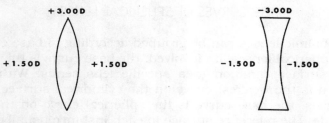

FIGURE 1.13   *Biconvex*   FIGURE 1.14   *Biconcave*

3. Periscopic

The periscopic lens features a base curve of 1.25D. If the total lens power is plus, the base curve is −1.25D located on the ocular surface. With minus power lenses the base curve is +1.25D and is found on the nonocular side. The power of the opposite surface is the curve that, when combined with +1.25D or −1.25D (Figures 1.15 and 1.16), gives the total lens power. With the exception of certain high-power prescriptions, the periscopic lens is rarely used today.

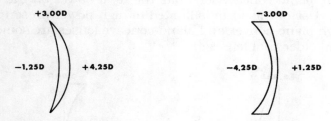

FIGURE 1.15   *Plus periscopic*   FIGURE 1.16   *Minus periscopic*

4. Meniscus

By convention, meniscus lenses have a base curve of 6.00D. However, any lens not of plano, biconvex, biconcave, periscopic, or corrected-curve form can be considered a meniscus lens. If the total power is plus, the base curve is always the ocular surface. The outside curve is that which, when combined with −6.00D (Figure 1.17), will give the desired power. With minus power lenses, the base curve is a plus curvature (usually +6.00D) (Figure 1.18) located on the outside surface. The meniscus lens is manufactured by many optical companies and is widely used in filling prescriptions.

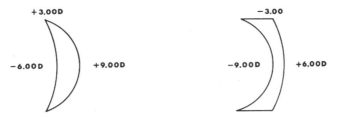

FIGURE 1.17   *Plus meniscus*   FIGURE 1.18   *Minus meniscus*

5. Corrected Curve

The base curve for each corrected lens varies according to the manufacturer, and the appropriate power chart must be consulted for specific values. While corrected lenses are designed to eliminate or reduce aberrations present in the peripheral portions of the lens, their importance is deemphasized with the fashion use of large-eye frames. It is impossible to eliminate peripheral distortion when oversize lenses are worn.

BASE CURVES OF CYLINDRICAL SINGLE-VISION LENSES

The base curve of a cylindrical lens is the weakest curve on the cylinder side. When the cylinder power is on the convex surface, the meridian having the least plus power is the base curve. For example, a lens $+1.00 + 2.00 \times 90°$ with an inside curve of $-6.00D$ has a base curve of $+7.00D$. This becomes evident by illustrating a side view of the lens with a cross line noting the cylindrical surface (Figure 1.19). The curves are designated as follows:

1.   The power on the concave surface is marked $-6.00D$.

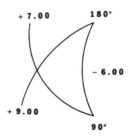

FIGURE 1.19

2. On the convex surface, the power in the meridian of the axis is +7.00D. It is the power that, when combined algebraically with the ocular surface (−6.00D), yields the spherical component of the prescription. For example, +7.00D + (−6.00D) = +1.00D.
3. The power of the curve 90° away from the axis is +9.00D. Because the axis is the meridian of least power, the cross curve manifests more plus power by the amount of the cylinder (i.e., +2.00D).
4. Because by definition the base curve is the weakest curve on the cylinder side, the base curve is +7.00D (meridian of least power).

When the cylinder is on the concave surface, the meridian having the least power is the base curve. For example (Figure 1.20), a lens +1.00 − 3.00 × 180° with an outside curve of +7.00D has a base curve of −6.00D.

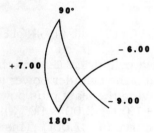

FIGURE 1.20

1. The power on the convex surface is +7.00D.
2. On the concave surface, the power in the meridian of the axis is −6.00D. When this power is combined algebraically with the nonocular surface (+7.00D), the result is the spherical component of the prescription, that is, +7.00D + (−6.00D) = +1.00D.
3. The power at 90° is −9.00D (cylinder difference of 3.00D).
4. The base curve is −6.00D (weakest curve on the cylinder side).

Note: Laboratories are also identifying the spherical outside curve of minus cylinder lenses as the base curve. Therefore, when ordering, the eyecare professional must be specific.

VERTEX DISTANCE AND ITS RELATION TO EFFECTIVE POWER

Emmetropia is that condition in which distant objects are focused clearly on the retina without the use of accommodation. The far point of the emmetropic eye is at infinity; that is, rays of light from infinity are conjugate with the retina (20 feet or more is considered optical infinity).

If a patient is not emmetropic (hyperopic, myopic, or astigmatic), correcting lenses must be placed in a certain position to allow parallel light entering the eye to focus on the retina. By common consent, manufacturers calculate the optics of lenses so that the power is true when the back surface of a lens is 13.75mm anterior to the cornea (vertex power). In practice, this distance is rarely measured because the discrepancy of a few millimeters normally does not make a significant difference in visual acuity.

However, when a high-power prescription is involved, vertex distance is critical and should be measured to determine the *effective power* of the lens. Effective power is defined as the vergence power of an optical system with respect to a particular reference point other than the principal point. In practice, the retina of the eye is usually designated as the reference plane and lens effectivity determined accordingly. The primary concern is alteration in effectivity when a high-power lens is moved closer to or farther from the eye (i.e., as the vertex distance is changed). Moving a convex lens away from the eye increases its effective power because the image is now formed in front of the retina; consequently, a weaker plus lens may have to be prescribed. Conversely, moving a concave lens away from the eye reduces its effectivity since the image is now theoretically formed behind the retina.

The change in effectivity as the vertex distance is altered is calculated with the following formula:

$$F_{\text{effective power}} = \frac{F_{\text{true power}}}{1 - dF_{\text{true power}}}$$

$F_{\text{true power}}$ refers to the actual power of the lens as determined by the focal length; $F_{\text{effective power}}$ refers to the lens power with respect to the retina (the reference plane). The distance in meters that the lens is moved from its original position is indicated by the letter *d*.

PROBLEM:

A +10.00D lens that forms a clear image on the retina is moved 5mm farther from the eye. Compute the effective power in this new position.

SOLUTION:

$$F_{\text{effective power}} = \frac{F_{\text{true power}}}{1 - dF_{\text{true power}}}$$

$$= \frac{+10.00}{1 - (0.005)(10)}$$

$$= +10.53D$$

PROBLEM:

A patient is refracted 10mm anterior to his corneal vertex. He is found to need a −10.00D lens in front of each eye. If his glasses are worn 15mm anterior to the corneal vertex, what is the effective power in this position?

SOLUTION:

$$F_{\text{eff}} = \frac{F_{\text{true}}}{1 - dF_{\text{true}}}$$

$$= \frac{-10.00}{1 - (0.005)(-10)}$$

$$= -9.50D$$

ABERRATIONS OF LENSES

Lens aberrations result when rays from a point source fail to form a perfect point image after traversing an optical system. All ophthalmic lenses have certain aberrations. One, chromatic aberration, derives from the nature of glass; the other five— spherical aberration, coma, marginal or oblique astigmatism, curvature of field, and distortion—are a result of the lens design. Some of these aberrations may be reduced; in essence, this is the purpose of corrected-curve lenses. However, it is important to recognize that the use of oversize blanks for certain frame designs must invalidate some of the applications of corrected-curve lenses.

1. Chromatic Aberration

Chromatic aberration results from the splitting of white light into component spectral colors when it is refracted by a glass lens (Figure 1.21). Because each wavelength has a different speed in any medium heavier than air, glass has a different refractive index for the various wavelengths.

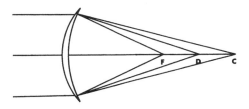

FIGURE 1.21   *Chromatic aberration*

This dispersive property manifests itself by focusing the blue, or F, line of the spectrum before the yellow, or D, line; the red of the C line focuses after the D.

Note: The power of a lens is arbitrarily determined by the focus of the D (yellow) line of the Fraunhofer spectrum. These lines denote particular colors of the spectrum, each occupying a constant position corresponding to a specific wavelength.

Although chromatic aberration can be corrected by combining two thin lenses of different indices to obtain an achromatic doublet, this aberration is not considered serious. Single-vision lenses manufactured of crown glass have a relatively low dispersive value. Also, the eye itself is not achromatic.

2. Spherical Aberration

Spherical aberration results because different zones of a lens have different powers (Figure 1.22). Peripheral and paraxial rays focus at different points along the axis, but because the pupil acts to limit the number of rays entering the eye, spherical aberration is not an ophthalmic problem.

3. Coma

Coma occurs because different areas of a lens project images of different size (Figure 1.23). An image of a point off the optical axis appears comet-shaped with the tail pointing toward the axis. Coma is not a concern in ophthalmic lenses because the pupil acts as an aperture to eliminate the peripheral rays.

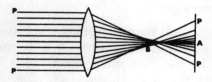

FIGURE 1.22   *Spherical aberration*

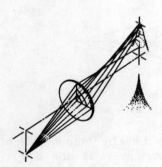

FIGURE 1.23   *Coma*

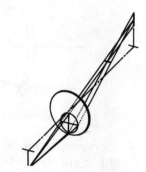

FIGURE 1.24   *Marginal astigmatism*

4. Marginal Astigmatism (Also Known as Radial or Oblique Astigmatism)

Marginal astigmatism results when a small bundle of light strikes a lens from an oblique angle forming two line images of a point source (Figure 1.24). As a consequence, objects viewed obliquely through an ophthalmic lens may be blurred. Marginal astigmatism is often a source of discomfort to the patient, and its reduction is an objective of use of corrected-curve lenses. However, all large lenses (over 52mm horizontal box measurement) exhibit peripheral distortion that cannot be eliminated.

5. Curvature of Field (Also Called Curvature of the Image)

Lenses do not form images of objects in a flat plane at the focal distance. Instead, curved images are formed concave toward the lenses (Figure 1.25). This aberration results from each object point being a different distance from the refracting surface. Reduction or elimination of curvature of field is another goal of corrected-curve lenses.

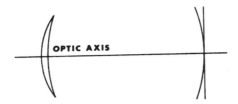

FIGURE 1.25   *Curvature of field*

6. Distortion

Distortion results from unequal magnification of object points not on the optical axis of a lens (Figure 1.26). When a patient looks through the periphery of a lens, the image is not in true proportion to the object. Through plus lenses, the image of a square has a pincushion appearance because the corners appear farther from the center than expected. When minus lenses are involved, the square appears barrel-shaped because the corners of the image seem closer to the center. Although lens curvatures designed to eliminate marginal astigmatism also reduce distortion, it is still necessary for patients to adjust to some effects of this aberration. There is apparent motion of objects when the head is turned, particularly with high power prescriptions. In addition, straight lines may appear curved, and curved objects distorted.

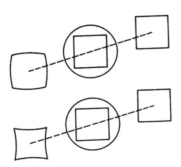

FIGURE 1.26   *Distortion*

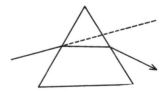

FIGURE 1.27   *Prism*

PRISM PRESCRIPTIONS

Prism prescriptions can be written independently or incorporated into a spherical, cylindrical, or sphero-cylinder correction. A prism lens does not converge or diverge light but instead deviates the rays passing through it. In certain cases, binocular vision cannot be achieved without this type of correction; in others, the patient is more comfortable when prisms are worn.

A prism is constructed with an apex (a thin edge) and a base (Figure 1.27). Light is deviated toward the base with the image projected in the direction of the apex. The unit of measurement is the prism diopter, indicated by the exponent ᐃ. One prism diopter deviates light 1cm at a distance of 1m on a tangent scale. This unit was suggested by Prentice (about 1890) because of its simplicity in computing and recording prism power.

PRISM EFFECTS IN A LENS

A prismatic effect is created when the patient looks away from the optical center of any plus or minus lens (Figures 1.28 and 1.29). This is easily visualized by noting that a convex lens may be considered a group of prisms with the bases touching at the center; conversely, a minus lens has its apexes coinciding at the center.

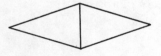

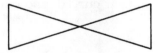

FIGURE 1.28 *Plus lens*   FIGURE 1.29 *Minus lens*

If the patient looks away from the lens center, the effect is that of a prism with its base in, out, up, or down, depending upon the direction of the gaze and the power of the lens. Prismatic effect can be computed by applying Prentice's law:

Prismatic effect = Lens power × Decentration (in centimeters)

Decentration is the distance from the center of the lens to the point in question. This distance is normally measured in millimeters and therefore must be converted to centimeters before the above formula is applied.

PROBLEM:

Given a +5.00D lens, find the prismatic effect when the patient looks 15mm nasal to the optical center.

SOLUTION:

$$\text{Prismatic effect} = F \times \text{decentration}$$
$$= +5.00 \times 1^1/_2\text{cm}$$
$$= 7^1/_2^\Delta \text{ base out}$$

PROBLEM:

Given a −8.00 lens, find the prismatic effect when the patient looks 12mm below the optical center.

SOLUTION:

$$\text{Prismatic effect} = F \times \text{decentration}$$
$$= -8.00 \times 1.2\text{cm}$$
$$= 9.6^\Delta \text{ base down}$$

When prism is to be incorporated into a prescription, sometimes it may be ordered by indicating the amount and direction of decentration. This is feasible only if the lens power is high enough and the lens blank of adequate size. When in doubt, query the laboratory.

PRISMATIC EFFECT WHEN TWO PRISMS ARE COMBINED

It is possible that the practitioner may want to know the combined effect of two prisms. This is determined by graphing the involved prismatic powers as illustrated in the following problems.

PROBLEM:

What is the resultant effect when the following prisms are combined?

$$2^\Delta \text{ base up at } 20°$$
$$5^\Delta \text{ base up at } 70°$$

PROCEDURE:

1.   The prismatic powers are graphed along an A line and a B line. Prism A is the one whose position is closest to the numerical value zero.

$$\text{A prism} = 2^\Delta \text{ base up}$$
$$\text{B prism} = 5^\Delta \text{ base up}$$

2. Prism A is plotted on the base line. Prism B is constructed α degrees away. α is the difference between the two axes.

$$70° - 20° = 50°$$

3. Graph prism A and prism B separated by α (50°). Complete the parallelogram (Figure 1.30). Draw the dotted line R from the point of origin to the opposite extremity of the parallelogram.

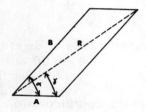

FIGURE 1.30

4. The dotted line R represents the prismatic effect. Measured R = $6^{1}/2^{\Delta}$.

5. The base positioning is determined by adding the position of A to γ. γ is the angle between A and R. γ = $36^{1}/2°$. The base positioning is $56^{1}/2°$ ($20°$ + $36^{1}/2°$).

SOLUTION:

Resultant prism = $6^{1}/2^{\Delta}$ base up at $56^{1}/2°$.

PROBLEM:

6^{Δ} base down at $10°$
5^{Δ} base down at $25°$

PROCEDURE:

1. Prism A is 6^{Δ} (positioned closest to numerical value zero). Prism B is 5^{Δ}.
2. α = $25° - 10° = 15°$
3. Graph prism A and prism B separated by α ($15°$) (Figure 1.31).
4. Measured R = 11^{Δ}

5. $\gamma = 7°$ (angle between A and R) γ, added to the positioning of prism A, $= 17°$ ($10° + 7°$).

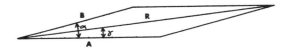

FIGURE 1.31

SOLUTION:

Resultant prism $= 11^\Delta$ base down at $17°$.

MEASUREMENT OF LENS AND/OR PRISM POWER

It is often necessary for the practitioner to determine the power of a lens prescription and/or whether a prism correction has been incorporated. For example, if glasses have been worn, the dioptric and/or prism power has to be ascertained before a new prescription is written. In addition, all prescriptions ordered from the laboratory must be checked for accuracy before the lenses are dispensed to the patient.

It is customary to determine a lens prescription and/or the amount of prism incorporated by the use of a lensometer or vertexometer. The optical system of these instruments is such that it is possible to read the prescription directly from the dials after focusing the target. Each instrument has the manufacturer's instructions for its use.

There are two other methods of determining lens prescriptions, although rarely is either used for this purpose. One is hand neutralization and the other is the use of a lens gauge.

Instructions for Hand Neutralization

If the lens power is outside the limits of the lensometer, hand neutralization may be employed. Hand neutralization involves using a lens of known power to neutralize the motion seen through the lens of unknown power. It will be remembered that characteristically a lens of zero power demonstrates no motion, a spherical lens of plus power exhibits *against motion,* and a minus spherical lens displays "with motion." A sphero-cylinder has different powers in the two principal meridians; therefore, the observed motion is neutralized by two different lenses corresponding to these meridians.

The lens to be neutralized must first be checked to see whether it is a sphere, cylinder, or sphere-cylinder. The observer holds the lens at arm's length and views a line object, such as the straight edge of a door or window. If the rotation produces a break in the continuity of the line, the lens is a cylinder or a sphero-cylinder; if there is no break, the lens is spherical. If against motion is noted, the unknown lens is of plus power, and a minus lens is arbitrarily selected from the trial lens case for neutralization. By trial and error this process is repeated until both lenses placed together produce no motion. If the unknown lens shows with motion, the lens is minus power, and plus lenses are selected for neutralization. In hand neutralizing sphero-cylinders, the two principal meridians are neutralized independently and the powers recorded on the optical cross. The prescription is then recorded as crossed cylinders and transposed into plus or minus cylinder form.

Note: The power of spherical, high plus lenses also can be found by means of holding the lens in front of an object and determining the best focus. Because the distance from the object to the lens is the focal length, its power is easily calculated.

Determining Lens Power with the Lens Gauge

Lens power can be ascertained by use of a lens gauge (sometimes referred to as a lens clock). This hand-held gauge, about 2 inches in diameter, is circular and has two outer fixed prongs with a movable pin between them. On the face of the clock are two concentric circles having numbers that indicate dioptric values. The black values of the inner circle denote the power of the convex surface of the lens; the red numbers of the outer circle give the power of the concave surface. In determining the lens power, the prongs of the clock are placed perpendicularly on the lens surface.

If the hand does not move when the clock is rotated on either surface, the lens is spherical. The readings of both surfaces are added algebraically to give the approximate power of the lens (thickness is not taken into consideration).

If the hand on the face of the clock moves, the surface is cylindrical, the amount of cylinder being the difference between the highest and lowest readings. For example, if the hand moves from 7.00D to 9.00D and with further rotation back toward 7.00D, the cylinder is 2.00D. If this movement is observed on the convex surface, a plus cylinder is involved; if on the concave surface, a minus cylinder is involved. Because the axis and the meridian of maximum power are 90° apart, the clock must be turned through an angle of 90° to determine the maximum and minimal readings. To determine the prescription, the powers in the two principal meridians are each algebraically combined with the spherical power of the opposite surface.

For example, the clock reading for the concave lens surface is −7.00D. The convex surface reads +7.00D in the 90° meridian and +8.00D in the 180°. Therefore, the prescription is Plano + 1.00 × 90°.

From a practical viewpoint, lens clocks are used only to determine the curvature of a particular surface and/or to ascertain the cylinder design. The practitioner usually checks the curves of the lenses the patient is wearing. If wishing to prescribe the same lens form or use other specific lens designs, the lens clock is utilized to confirm laboratory accuracy. It is also used to check bitoric effects (cylinder on both surfaces) of plastic lenses after they are mounted (see Chapter 7, "Plastic Ophthalmic Lenses").

Lens gauges are calibrated for an index of 1.53. If the lens is manufactured of plastic or of glass having another index, the approximate power must be determined. The conversation formula is as follows:

$$F = R\left(\frac{n-1}{c-1}\right)$$

F = true power of the lens
R = reading on the lens gauge
n = index of the lens
c = index for which the clock is calibrated

PROBLEM:

The total power of a lens as determined with a lens gauge is +6.00D.
Find the true power if the index of the lens is 1.60.

SOLUTION:

$$F_{true} = R\left(\frac{n-1}{c-1}\right)$$

$$= +6.00D\left(\frac{1.60-1}{1.53-1}\right)$$

$$= +6.80D$$

PROBLEM:

The total power of a lens as determined with a lens gauge is −4.50D.
Find the true power if the index of the lens is 1.47.

SOLUTION:

$$F_{true} = R\left(\frac{n-1}{c-1}\right)$$

$$= -4.50D\left(\frac{1.47-1}{1.53-1}\right)$$

$$= -3.96D$$

PROBLEM:

If the true power of a lens of index 1.50 is +5.00D, what is the lens gauge reading?

SOLUTION:

$$F_{true} = R\left(\frac{n-1}{c-1}\right)$$

$$+5.00 = R\left(\frac{1.50-1}{1.53-1}\right)$$

$$R = +5.30D$$

PROBLEM:

If a −4.00D lens has a lens gauge reading of −4.25D, what is the index of the lens?

SOLUTION:

$$F_{true} = R\left(\frac{n-1}{c-1}\right)$$

$$-4.00 = -4.25\left(\frac{n-1}{153-1}\right)$$

$$(n-1) = 0.457$$

$$n = 1.47$$

Chapter 2

INTRODUCTION TO BIFOCAL LENSES

HISTORY OF BIFOCAL LENSES

A bifocal lens is an ingenious device having two focal lengths in one lens. It is used primarily for the correction of presbyopia (the technical term for the diminishing plasticity of the crystalline lens). This condition necessitates additional plus power at near and usually becomes critical in the midforties. Bifocals are also used in cases of muscle imbalance in which the patient needs more plus at near for comfortable vision.

Benjamin Franklin invented the bifocal lens to eliminate the inconvenience of using separate pairs of glasses for distance and near. The solution seems so logical, it is surprising that this lens form did not appear until 1784. The original Franklin bifocal featured a halved distance lens and a halved near correction placed in juxtaposition and held together by a circular metal-rimmed frame. The principle behind this split bifocal is seen in the modern straight-across design.

It was inevitable that the convenience and practical value of a multifocal lens design would result in improved versions. The first one-piece bifocal (change in power for near achieved through a change in curvature of one surface) appeared to have its beginning in 1837. Called the Solid Upcurve Bifocal, it was patented by Isaac Schnaitman of Philadelphia and was manufactured so that the top portion of a biconvex lens was ground flat on one surface. The finished lens was, therefore, a combination of a plano-convex and a biconvex lens.

Two more bifocal designs were patented in 1888 by August Marich. One, known as the Perfection Bifocal, had the same basic principle as the Benjamin Franklin split bifocal. Two separate pieces of crown glass were utilized, the segment area being semicircular in appearance. The other bifocal featured a crown glass major lens to which was cemented a "wafer" of spherical power equivalent to the near add. It was known as the Cement Bifocal. Canada balsam, the adhesive used, presented many problems. Under warm conditions the segment tended to slide; in cold weather the wafer would sometimes break away from the major lens. In addition, regardless of how skilled the optician was in cementing the segment, aberrations were present that interfered with clarity of vision. Later another cement lens, known as Opifex Bifocal, was introduced. It somewhat improved upon the original design, but the obvious disadvantages of using cement to attach the plus power wafer were still present.

The first attempt at gaining additional power at near by using a glass button of a higher index of refraction was made by John Borsch, Sr., in 1899. A countersink curve was formed on the convex surface of the major blank into which was cemented a small flint segment. In the final step of manufacture, a cover lens of crown glass was cemented over the entire front surface of the lens. This bifocal design was called the Kryptok lens, named after the Greek word *kryptos* meaning "hidden."

In 1908 John Borsch, Jr., invented the first fused bifocal, retaining the name of his father's original lens design, Kryptok. A round segment button was fused into a major blank that had been prepared by removing a section into which the higher index segment could be fused. The near power was controlled by the ratio of the two indices and the radius of the countersink curve.

The first one-piece bifocals to be available widely were manufactured in 1910 by Continental Optical Co. The lens series was distributed under the trade name Ultex and is still produced today.

In 1926, the bifocal that has been the most popular to date was introduced by Univis Lens Co. Of fused construction, it featured a straight dividing line, which eliminated the superfluous upper area of the round segment. This resulted in an optical center located closer to the top of the segment, thereby reducing the amount of image jump. Since its introduction, it has been copied with minor modifications by every major lens manufacturer.

The next bifocal that proved extremely successful was a one-piece straight-across design similar in appearance to the original Benjamin Franklin split bifocal. Introduced by American Optical Corp. in the late 1950s, it is distributed under the trade name Executive.

Although bifocal lenses enabled a presbyope the convenience of clear, near vision without changing glasses, some patients objected to the appearance of the dividing line, feeling it was a telltale sign of maturity. As a result, lens manufacturers attempted to produce a bifocal without a dividing line. The first relatively successful effort was the Younger Seamless bifocal designed in the middle 1950s. The sharp line of demarcation of conventional bifocals was polished out. However, it had its drawbacks in that this blending resulted in a blurred area with an uncontrollable cylindrical power at an oblique axis.

MODERN BIFOCAL DESIGNS

There are two basic forms of construction used in the manufacture of contemporary bifocals. The fused bifocal features a crown glass major lens blank, usually of 1.523 index, for the distance correction. The near prescription is obtained by fusing a segment of higher index into a designated countersink curve in the major blank. Most quality bifocal manufacturers prefer barium segments whenever possible because the low dispersion factor and relative hardness make this a practical type of segment glass. However, flint glass is sometimes combined with barium to give the higher index of refraction necessary for certain segment powers.

The other basic bifocal design features a one-piece form of construction. The change in near power results from a change in curvature on one surface of the lens. All bifocals utilizing a high-index glass for a distance correction and all bifocals made of plastic are of a one-piece construction. Some one-piece designs are available in crown glass.

One-piece bifocals, with the exception of the seamless (blended) design, can be identified by a ridge that divides the distance correction from the near. It is felt by moving a finger across the segment side of the lens. Because a fused bifocal has a button designed to fit the countersink curve and the spherical curve of the segment is the same as the distance correction, a ridge is not present.

TYPES OF BIFOCAL DESIGNS

Fused and one-piece bifocal lenses of contemporary design are further subdivided into five basic types. The classifications are determined by the shape of the segment:

1.   Round-top bifocals
2.   Straight-top bifocals
3.   Curved-top bifocals
4.   Straight-across bifocals
5.   "Invisible" bifocals

1. Round-top Bifocals

The round-top bifocal is constructed in such a manner that the segment forms a perfect circle. However, when the lenses are cut to fit the frame, the segments are almost always semicircular in shape. Round-top bifocals are produced in both fused and one-piece designs. By the nature of the construction, the optical center of the segment is the exact center of the original round button.

2. Straight-top Bifocals (Also Known as Flat-top Bifocals)

Lenses that fall into this category feature a straight-line division that does not extend to either the nasal or temporal extremity in the factory blank. However, when the bifocal lens is cut and edged to fit a specific frame, it is possible, although unusual, that the segment line may reach one or both edges of the lens. These lenses may be fused or one-piece in construction.

The majority of straight-top bifocals feature segments with upper corners that are sharply outlined; some are manufactured with the upper limits rounded in shape. The most often prescribed are designed in such a manner that the lower edge of the segment forms a semicircular pattern. A limited few feature straight lines for both upper and lower extremities.

Almost since its introduction, the straight-top bifocal has been the most popular of the modern multifocal designs. The relatively useless upper area of the round-top segment is eliminated, allowing patients to hold their heads in a more normal position when using the widest area of the segment.

3. Curved-top Bifocals

This category consists of bifocals featuring a curved dividing line with the lower segment edge always circular in shape. The outer limits of the dividing line are either sharp or rounded, depending on the particular design.

4. Straight-across Bifocals

This bifocal design is always a one-piece construction. The dividing line is an inverted "shelf" extending from the nasal to the temporal edges of the nonocular surface of the lens. This multifocal design is a sophisticated version of the original Benjamin Franklin split bifocal. It features the "no jump" principle since the optical centers of the distance and near prescriptions are at the dividing line.

5. "Invisible" Bifocal Designs

The seamless (blended) are the bifocal designs in this category. They are discussed in Chapter 5, "Prescribing 'Invisible' Multifocals."

MATHEMATICAL COMPUTATIONS INVOLVING FUSED BIFOCALS

To understand bifocal design better, some of the mathematical calculations involved in determining the specifications for proper adds in bifocal corrections are given.

The dioptric power of the add of a fused bifocal is determined by the relationship of the index of the glass used in the distance correction and the higher index of the glass used in the near portion. These indices, in turn, determine the power of the countersink curve needed to give the additional dioptric power in the segment (Figure 2.1).

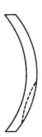

FIGURE 2.1 *Countersink curve*

The formulas used in these calculations are as follows:

$$F_i = \frac{n_n - 1}{n_d - 1} \times F_{front}$$

F_i = power change caused by the change in indices
n_n = index of the near add
n_d = index of the distance correction
F_{front} = dioptric curvature of the front surface

$$F_{gain} = F_i - F_{front}$$

F_{gain} = power gained by the change in indices
F_i = power change caused by the change in indices
F_{front} = dioptric curvature of the front surface

$$F_{needed} = F_{add} - F_{gain}$$

F_{needed} = additional power to give total power of the segment
F_{add} = total add power
F_{gain} = power gained by the change in indices

$$r = \frac{n_d - n_n}{F_{needed}}$$

r = radius of the countersink curve in meters
n_d = index of the distance correction
n_n = index of the near add
F_{needed} = additional power needed to give total power of the segment

$$F_{cc}\ \frac{n_d - 1}{r}$$

F_{cc} = dioptric power of the countersink curve
n_d = index of the distance correction
r = radius of the countersink curve

$$F_{rf} = F_{ocular} + F_{cc}$$

F_{rf} = dioptric power of reading field

F_{ocular} = dioptric power of ocular surface of the lens

F_{cc} = dioptric power of countersink curve

PROBLEM:

A round-top fused bifocal has a distance power of +6.00D; the add is +3.00D. The inside of the lens is −8.00D. The distance index is 1.523; the near index is 1.62. Find the following:

(a) the radius of the countersink curve
(b) the power of the countersink curve
(c) the power of the reading field before fusing

PROCEDURE FOR (a):

1. Determine the power change caused by the change in indices.

$$F_I = \frac{n_n - 1}{n_d - 1} \times F_{front}$$

$$= \frac{1.62 - 1}{1.523 - 1} \times 14$$

$$= 16.6D$$

2. Determine the power gained because of the index.

$$F_{gain} = F_i - F_{front}$$

$$= 16.6 - 14.0$$

$$= 2.6D$$

3. Determine the power needed.

$$F_{needed} = F_{add} - F_{gain}$$

$$= 3.00 - 2.60$$

$$= 0.40D$$

4.   Determine the radius of the countersink curve.

$$r = \frac{n_d - n_n}{F_{needed}}$$

$$= \frac{1.523 - 1.62}{0.40}$$

$$= -0.24m$$

Solution to (a):

Countersink curve radius = − 0.24m

Procedure for (b):

Determine the power of the countersink curve.

$$F_{cc} = \frac{n_d - 1}{r}$$

$$= \frac{1.523 - 1}{-0.24}$$

$$= -2.18D$$

Solution to (b):

Countersink curve power = −2.18D

Procedure for (c):

Determine the power of the reading field before fusing.

$$F_{rf} = F_{ocular} + F_{cc}$$
$$= -8.00 + (-2.18)$$
$$= -10.18D$$

Solution to (c):

Power of the reading field before fusing = − 10.18D

PROBLEM:

A round-top fused bifocal has a distance power of $-4.00D$; the add is $+2.00D$. The inside curve of the lens is $-10.00D$. The near index is 1.60. Find the following:
(a) the radius of the countersink curve
(b) the power of the countersink curve
(c) the power of the reading field before fusing
(d) the thickness of the button
Assume the distance index is 1.523 and the segment is a 22mm round.

PROCEDURE FOR (a):

1. Determine the power change caused by the index.

$$F_I = \frac{n_n - 1}{n_d - 1} \times F_{front}$$

$$= \frac{1.60 - 1}{1.523 - 1} \times 6$$

$$= 6.90D$$

2. Determine the power gained because of the index.

$$F_{gain} = F_i - F_{front}$$

$$= 6.9 - 6.0$$

$$= 0.9D$$

3. Determine the power needed.

$$F_{needed} = F_{add} - F_{gain}$$

$$= +2.00 - 0.9$$

$$= +1.10D$$

4. Determine the radius of the countersink curve.

$$r = \frac{n_d - n_n}{F_{needed}}$$

$$= \frac{1.523 - 1.6}{1.10}$$

$$= -0.07\text{m}$$

SOLUTION TO (a):

Countersink curve radius −0.07m

PROCEDURE FOR (b):

Determine the power of the countersink curve.

$$F_{cc} = \frac{n_d - 1}{r}$$

$$= \frac{1.523 - 1}{-0.07}$$

$$= 7.50\text{D}$$

SOLUTION TO (b):

Power of the countersink curve = −7.50D

PROCEDURE FOR (c):

Determine the power of the reading field before fusing.

$$F_{rf} = F_{ocular} + F_{cc}$$

$$= -10.00 + (-7.5)$$

$$= -17.50\text{D}$$

SOLUTION TO (c):

Power of the reading field before fusing = −17.50D

PROCEDURE FOR (d):

Determine the thickness of the button using the sagittal (thickness) formula.

$$Sag = \frac{(F_{front} - F_{cc})(\frac{1}{2} \text{ seg diameter})^2}{2(n_d - 1)}$$

$$= \frac{13.5(.011)^2}{2(1.523 - 1)}$$

$$= .0016m = 1.6mm$$

SOLUTION TO (d):

Thickness of the button = 1.6mm

PROBLEM:

A 22mm round-segment bifocal has a distance prescription of $+4.00 - 1.00 \times 45$, add $+3.50D$. The index of the distance portion is 1.523, and the index of the segment is 1.6. The inside curve of the lens is $-5.00D$. Find the following:
(a) the radius of the countersink curve
(b) the power of the countersink curve
(c) the power of the reading field before fusing
(d) the Kryptok factor (factory term for dioptric change in countersink curve that increases add by 1 diopter)
(e) the thickness of the button

PROCEDURE FOR (a):

1. Determine the power change caused by the change in indices.

Note: Since fused bifocals are manufactured in minus cylinder form, the cylinder is on the back surface and not taken into consideration when determining F_{front} curvature. If the prescription is written in plus cylinder form, transpose to minus using the new written correction to determine F_{front} (outside curvature).

$$Fi = \frac{n_n - 1}{n_d - 1} \times F_{front}$$

$$= \frac{1.60 - 1}{1.523 - 1} \times 9$$

$$= +10.33D$$

2.   Determine the power gained because of the index.

$$F_{gain} = F_i - F_{front}$$
$$= +10.33 - 9.00$$
$$= +1.33D$$

3.   Determine the power needed.

$$F_{needed} = F_{add} - F_{gain}$$
$$= +3.50 - (+1.33)$$
$$= +2.17D$$

4. Determine the radius of the countersink curve.

$$r = \frac{n_d - n_n}{F_{needed}}$$
$$= \frac{1.523 - 1.6}{+2.17}$$
$$= -0.0355m$$

SOLUTION TO (a):

Countersink curve radius = −0.0355m

PROCEDURE FOR (b):

Determine the power of the countersink curve.

$$F_{cc} = \frac{n_d - 1}{r}$$
$$= \frac{1.523 - 1}{-0.0355}$$
$$= -14.73D$$

SOLUTION TO (b):

Countersink curve power $= -14.73D$

PROCEDURE FOR (c):

Determine the power of the reading field before fusing.

$$F_{rf} = F_{ocular} + F_{cc}$$
$$= -5.00 + (-14.73)$$
$$= -19.73D$$

SOLUTION TO (c):

Power of the reading field before fusing $= -19.73D$

PROCEDURE FOR (d):

Determine the Kryptok factor (term remains by common usage).

$$K_f = \frac{n_d - 1}{n_n - n_d}$$
$$= \frac{1.523 - 1.00}{1.60 - 1.523}$$
$$= 6.79$$

SOLUTION TO (d):

Kryptok factor $= 6.79$

PROCEDURE FOR (e):

Determine the thickness of the segment button.

$$t = \frac{(F_{front} - F_{cc})\, h^2}{2(n_d - 1)}$$
$$= \frac{[+9.00 - (-14.73)](0.011)^2}{2(1.523 - 1)}$$
$$= 0.00275m = 2.75mm$$

SOLUTION TO (e):

Segment button thickness = 2.75mm

PROBLEM:

A round-top 24mm bifocal has a distance power of −5.00 −1.50 × 10. The add is +3.00D. The inside curve of the lens is −8.00D. The index of the distance portion of the lens is 1.5, and the index of the segment is 1.6. Find the following:
(a) the radius of the countersink curve
(b) the power of the countersink curve
(c) the power of the reading field before fusing
(d) the Kryptok factor (the term remains by common usage)
(e) the thickness of the button

PROCEDURE FOR (a):

1. Determine the power change caused by the change in indices.

$$F_I = \frac{n_n - 1}{n_d - 1} \times F_{front}$$

$$= \frac{1.6 - 1}{1.5 - 1} \times 3$$

$$= 3.6D$$

2. Determine the power gained because of the index.

$$F_{gain} = F_i - F_{front}$$

$$= 3.6 - 3.0$$

$$= 0.60D$$

3. Determine the power needed.

$$F_{needed} = F_{add} - F_{gain}$$

$$= 3.0 - 0.60$$

$$= 2.40D$$

4. Determine the radius of the countersink curve.

$$r = \frac{n_d - n_n}{F_{needed}}$$
$$= \frac{1.5 - 1.6}{2.4}$$
$$= -0.0417m$$

SOLUTION TO (a):

Countersink curve radius $= -0.0417m$

PROCEDURE FOR (b):

Determine the power of the countersink curve.

$$F_{cc} = \frac{n_d - 1}{r}$$
$$= \frac{1.5 - 1}{-0.0417}$$
$$= -12.00D$$

SOLUTION TO (b):

Countersink curve power $= -12.00D$

PROCEDURE FOR (c):

Determine the power of the reading field before fusing.

$$F_{rf} = F_{ocular} + F_{cc}$$
$$= -8.00 + (-12.00)$$
$$= -20.00D$$

SOLUTION TO (c):

Reading field power before fusing $= -20.00D$

PROCEDURE FOR (d):

Determine the Kryptok factor.

$$K_f = \frac{n_d - 1}{n_n - n_d}$$

$$= \frac{1.5 - 1}{1.6 - 1.5}$$

$$= 5$$

SOLUTION TO (d):

Kryptok factor = 5 (term remains by common usage)

PROCEDURE FOR (e):

Determine the thickness of the segment button.

$$t = \frac{(F_{front} - F_{cc})h^2}{2(n_d - 1)}$$

$$= \frac{[3.00 - (-12.00)](0.012)^2}{2(1.5 - 1)}$$

$$= 0.0022m = 2.2mm$$

SOLUTION TO (e):

Segment button thickness = 2.2mm

PRESCRIBING MODERN GLASS BIFOCAL DESIGNS

INTRODUCTION

Contemporary bifocal lenses intended for general-purpose wear or prescribed for vocational/avocational purposes are available to fill the needs of every patient requiring such a correction. Popular designs are manufactured in both glass and plastic. While it is highly recommended that whenever possible plastic rather than glass lenses be prescribed, there are certain bifocals available only in glass. This chapter concerns itself with conventional glass bifocals. Chapter 7, "Plastic Ophthalmic Lenses," analyzes the hard resin (CR 39) plastic designs, polycarbonate, and other high-index plastic lenses.

Lenses are illustrated with explanations for prescribing considerations; trade names are used when the particular design is identified with its creator and/or its distributor. Lenses that may no longer be available are included because patients may still be wearing the bifocal and need to be prescribed another design.

Note: Bifocals manufactured in special forms, such as photochromic and cataract lenses, are covered in the chapters involving those areas: Chapter 9, "Prescribing Absorptive Lenses," and Chapter 11, "Lenses That Serve Special Needs."

Glass bifocals can have either a fused or a one-piece construction. (All plastic bifocals are one piece.) Fused glass bifocals manufactured in the United States are in minus cylinder form with the segment fused on the outside surface. The major blank is fashioned of crown glass, index 1.523; the segment is of a higher index, either barium or a combination of barium and flint. A very few are made of flint glass only. Flint causes more chromatic aberration than barium, so most manufacturers limit its content, although the higher index of refraction makes it a necessity for certain high-add lenses.

One-piece glass bifocals are either plus or minus cylinder form, although manufacturers in the United States have discontinued the plus-cylinder design. Almost all are fashioned of crown glass, index 1.523, except for a very few constructed of high-index glass. These are intended for strong minus corrections and are identified in the text. When a finger is run over the segment side of a one-piece bifocal, the ridge dividing the distance from the near area can be felt. This method is frequently used to distinguish fused bifocals from the one-piece designs.

Theoretically, one-piece bifocals fashioned of crown glass have less chromatic aberration and are lighter than the fused designs, which by necessity utilize the heavier barium and/or flint segments. Practically speaking, however, patients notice little difference, except, of course, in cases of high-index glass lenses. Therefore, the design recommended to the patient depends on its optical characteristics: position of segment optical center, width of segment, etc.

IMAGE JUMP VS. OBJECT DISPLACEMENT

At one time it was felt that a patient needing a bifocal with a plus distance correction should be prescribed a round-top design. The low placement of the segment optical center reduces or eliminates the base-up effect of the distance when viewing near objects. (Base up was neutralized by base down because the patient looked above the segment optical center when reading.) Today, practitioners feel the reduction of image jump as the patient's eye travels from distance to near is more critical. Since image jump is controlled by the segment optical center (the closer the optical center is to the dividing line, the less the image jump), contemporary bifocals of a straight-top design with an optical center 3 to 5mm below the dividing line are preferred for most prescriptions. (Lenses that have a segment optical center at the dividing line lack cosmetic appeal.) These bifocals allow the patient to hold the neck and head in relatively comfortable normal positions, because the widest part of the segment (through the optical center) is reached almost as soon as the line of sight passes into the add power.

STRAIGHT-TOP FUSED BIFOCAL SEGMENTS WITH SHARP CORNERS AND ROUNDED LOWER EXTREMITIES

These fused lenses produced by all major manufacturers are the most widely prescribed glass bifocals in the United States. The impractical upper area of a round segment button is eliminated, resulting in a segment optical center ranging from 3 to 5 mm below the dividing line (depending on the design), thus minimizing image jump.

There are several changes involving the manufacture of these lenses. Univis, Inc., who developed the design under the name Univis D, sold its lens division to Vision-Ease Lens in 1982–1983. This company retained only the *D* to identify the straight-top/flat-top series. Bausch & Lomb, Inc., who released the designs under the trade name Orthogon straight-top, no longer manufacturers multifocals. The lenses are currently distributed by all major manufacturers, but Vision-Ease Lens continues to be the major supplier. The lenses may also be identified as flat-top (FT) designs or straight-top (ST) in addition to D style. In the optical field the terms are interchangeable.

Flat Top 22 (22mm × 16mm), Also Identified as Straight Top (ST)

At one time, this was a widely prescribed bifocal. However, the size is being phased out because the ST25mm and ST28mm are considered general-purpose bifocals that better fill the need for an adequate near field. (The original ST18mm, 19mm, and 20mm lenses have not been available for decades.)

Flat Top 25 (25mm × 17mm), Also Known as Straight Top (ST)

This bifocal was originally intended as a compromise general-purpose and occupational lens for patients requiring a relatively large segment. The increase in occupations involving a great deal of close work has emphasized the importance of the ST25mm. It is usually recommended for first-time bifocal wearers and is almost always used to replace the ST22mm when the patient needs a new bifocal correction. The segment optical center is 5mm below the dividing line (Figure 3.1).

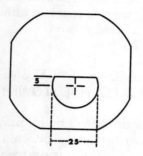

FIGURE 3.1   *Flat top 25*

Flat Top 28 (28mm × 19mm), Also Identified as Straight Top (ST)

The ST28mm was designed as an occupational lens for patients requiring a large segment area. It was recommended only for accountants, teachers, secretaries, and others involved in many hours of near work. In view of the comfort it affords, today practitioners often prescribe it as a general-purpose bifocal. Because the optical center is 5mm below the dividing line, the ST28mm can provide horizontal prism at the near point when such a need is indicated (Figure 3.2). Although the overdecentration results in a less usable near area, this method of obtaining prism at the reading level is superior both optically and cosmetically to a factory-ground prism segment.

Flat Top 35 (35mm × 22.5mm), Also Identified as Straight Top (ST)

The ST35 is usually limited to patients requiring an occupational bifocal. Like all large-segment lenses, its cosmetic appearance is not as pleasing as that of bifocals that utilize a smaller reading area. The dividing line becomes especially prominent when a high add is involved. Most manufacturers place the optical center 3mm below the dividing line (Figure 3.3), but there may be some variation. Check with the laboratory if this is a consideration.

Vision-Ease sets the optical center 5mm below the dividing line so the lens can be overdecentered to provide horizontal prism at the near point when such a need is indicated. The lens is identified as a D style, and Vision-Ease will compute the decentration for the practitioner. This method is superior both optically and cosmetically to a factory-ground prism segment and should be utilized if feasible.

Note: The ST45, a fused bifocal having a horizontal measurement of 45mm, has been discontinued. The ST35 is the widest available glass lens in this basic style.

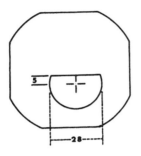

FIGURE 3.2   *Flat top 28*

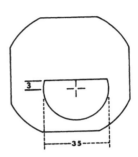

FIGURE 3.3   *Flat top 35*

Because of the great popularity of the flat top (straight top) designs, manufacturers make them available in a wide array of tints. Pink 1, 2, and 3; green 1, 2, and 3; gray 1 and 2; Photogray Extra and Photobrown Extra are almost always listed as standard tints in optical catalogues.

Note: Some straight top designs are no longer available, such as the Univis IS (identifiable segment), a 22mm flat-top glass bifocal with curved corners and rounded lower extremities. A similar-looking lens, Shuron-Continental's Ultex K one-piece bifocal, has not been manufactured for decades.

Straight Top Prism Segment (Vision-Ease)

There are patients who need a prism correction at near only. A possibility is the Vision-Ease Prism Segment. Calculations are programmed into a computer; the practitioner sends in the required prism amount (base in only is available), and calculations are done for the layout. The segment looks like a bar design (Figure 3.4). The vertical dimension is 10mm. The horizontal hovers around 22mm. Check with the laboratory for cost and time of delivery. It may be a better solution to provide the patient with the D-35 bifocal, decentered at near as much as possible, and a separate pair of near prescription lenses with the full needed prism correction.

Prism-segment bifocals are so rare that most practitioners have never seen them. There are reasons for not prescribing these lenses, as follows:

1. Cosmetic appearance: The segment looks like a miniature prism "tacked" onto a major lens and results in a unsightly, weird-looking design.
2. There is pronounced distortion through the segment as a result of the prism.
3. Color aberration: Patients see color fringes around reading material.
4. Near field of view is limited.

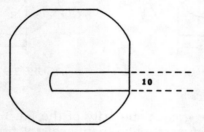

FIGURE 3.4   *Prism segment*

B Style Bar Segment (26mm × 9mm and 22mm × 9mm)

The B segment (meaning *bar*) has a long, narrow appearance. Although its horizontal size varies, 22mm or 26mm, the vertical remains a constant 9mm. The optical center is 4.5mm below the segment line, and the upper and lower divisions are straight lines of equal length (Figure 3.5). Its purpose is to give an injury-prone patient distant vision beneath the near area.

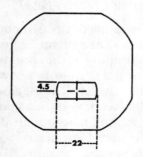

FIGURE 3.5   *Bar segment*

To accomplish this, the segment needs to be set at least 17mm high. These bifocals are rarely prescribed. If they are, it should be in conjunction with single-vision reading glasses. The segments are too small for prolonged pleasurable near viewing. (At one time, the B segment was available in 28mm × 9mm, but that size has long been discontinued.)

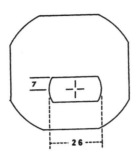

FIGURE 3.6 *R segment*

R Style (26mm × 14mm and 22mm × 14mm): The R Stands for Ribbon

The R-style (ribbon) segment should not be confused with the B style (bar) segment. The upper and lower limits of the R segment are straight lines of equal length, so they tend to look similar, but the R segment has an optical center 7mm below the dividing line (Figure 3.6). Originated by Univis and now available from Vision-Ease, the lens is rarely prescribed. The two division lines result in a prominent-looking bifocal, and the positioning of the optical center creates more image jump than a straight-top D-style segment.

Note: R-compensating bifocals (the standard R described above is no. 7 in the series) are available from Vision-Ease. However, their use is not a recommended method of compensating for vertical imbalance at the near point. Reasons are discussed in Chapter 13, "Vertical Imbalance at the Reading Level."

CURVE-TOP FUSED BIFOCALS WITH SHARP CORNERS

This design was developed by American Optical Corp. and originally distributed under the trade name Ful-Vue bifocal (later changed to Tillyer C and then to Tillyer Sovereign). It has the same basic optical properties as the straight-top D-style bifocal, although the segment features a slightly curved dividing line. Comparable lens designs in two sizes, called CXL 25 and CXL 28, are available from Vision-Ease Lens, but the flat-top (straight-top) designs serve the same purpose and have better cosmetic value.

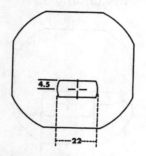

FIGURE 3.7   *Curve top 25*

Curve Top 25 (25mm × 17mm)

This size, originally considered a compromise general-purpose/occupational bifocal (Figure 3.7), functions in the same manner as the ST25mm design. However, the latter is more widely used because it has more cosmetic appeal. The optical center is 4mm below the segment dividing line.

Curve Top (28mm × 18.5mm)

The basic design of the Tillyer Sovereign is available in a 28mm horizontal size with an optical center 5mm below the dividing line. Prescribed as a large-segment, general-purpose lens, it can be used as the ST28mm bifocal is. However, the latter has a slightly less noticeable dividing line.

CURVED-TOP FUSED BIFOCALS WITH CURVED CORNERS: PANOPTIK (DISCONTINUED)

This design was originated by Bausch & Lomb under the trade name Orthogon Panoptik (Figure 3.8). It had a slightly curved dividing line with the upper segment extremities forming curved corners. The original Panoptik was widely advertised and available in two sizes: 22m × 14mm and 24mm × 16.5mm. The Panoptik style (now discontinued) was rarely prescribed for a number of years, and patients still wearing this design are best served with a D style, straight-top bifocal.

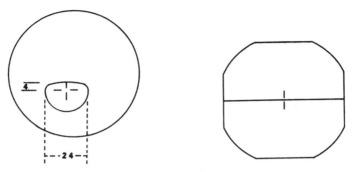

FIGURE 3.8 *Panoptik (discontinued)*   FIGURE 3.9 *Straight-across bifocal*

STRAIGHT-ACROSS (EXECUTIVE) BIFOCAL

The straight-across, minus cylinder, one-piece design was created by American Optical Corp. under the trade name Executive bifocal (Figure 3.9). It is distributed by many manufacturers and each local laboratory will supply the basic design of its provider. The Executive lens is considered an occupational bifocal. The segment extends from nasal to temporal extremities of the factory blank. Image jump is eliminated because the optical center is positioned at the dividing line. Laboratories are stressing that the Executive bifocal is not suitable for oversize frames. Although available in large blanks, the construction results in a relatively thick lens, making the glass version especially difficult to wear comfortably. The cosmetic disadvantage lies in the obvious inverted "shelves" located on the outside surface. These tend to chip, particularly when high-add glass designs are involved. The ST35mm may prove more satisfactory as an occupational bifocal.

ROUND-TOP FUSED BIFOCALS

Round-top bifocals are so called because the segments are a completed circle in the original factory blank. They almost always give the effect of a slightly full half-circle when cut to ordered segment height.

Some discontinued Bausch & Lomb trade names had become synonymous with round-top fused glass lenses: Orthogon C (16mm round), Orthogon D (20mm round), and Orthogon F (22mm round). Today, major manufacturers do not make a stock bifocal blank smaller than a 22mm round. However, fused round segments can be ground to a smaller diameter. For example, the round 16mm was originally intended as a golfer's bifocal set low in the finished lens so that the golfer could utilize the distance prescription without interference from the near correction. The size can still be ordered if desired, although it may not be listed in lens catalogues.

Note: Quality round-top 22mm bifocals are sometimes confused with the Kryptok lens available from numerous optical companies. The latter is designed to keep production costs at a minimum (manufacturers processing the Kryptok may not maintain the high standards required of quality lenses). In most cases, the type of glass used in the Kryptok segment causes high chromatic aberration that the patient sees as colored fringes around reading material.

ROUND-TOP 22 (22MM ROUND SEGMENT)

The round-top 22mm lens was originally designed as a general-purpose bifocal (Figure 3.10). However, positioning of the optical center (11mm below the segment line) results in considerable image jump as well as an uncomfortable head tilt when reaching the maximum near width. Today these lenses are prescribed only when the patient's primary concern is a cosmetic one. The segment is less visible than a straight-top or curved-top design. (In the lower adds, it is barely visible.) There are also patients who adapt more readily to and are more comfortable with the round-top bifocal because the change from distance to near is not exaggerated as with straight-top segment designs. The personality of the patient is the key factor in the recommendation of the round-top 22mm bifocal.

Round Top 25 (25mm Round Segment)

A 25mm round segment is listed as available from some manufacturers of glass lenses. The same considerations as for prescribing the round-top 22mm segments are in order. It must be remembered that a larger segment means it is slightly more visible.

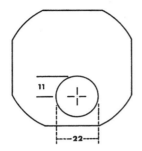

FIGURE 3.10 *Round-top 22*

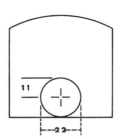

FIGURE 3.11 *Ultex B (discontinued)*

ROUND-TOP ONE-PIECE BIFOCALS

Ultex B (22mm Round, Discontinued)

Ultex B was the trade name for Shuron-Textron's 22mm round one-piece glass bifocal in plus cylinder form (Figure 3.11). The Orthogon B by Bausch & Lomb and the Tillyer B by American Optical were comparable lenses. This bifocal style was used for the same cases as a 22mm round-top fused design but is no longer available in the United States.

Ultex E (32mm × 16mm)

The Ultex E is semicircular and measures 32mm across at its widest point, which is the lowest extremity of the segment (Figure 3.12). In the manufacturing process, one large blank with a 32mm round segment is split through the center. The result is two lenses, each having an optical center 16mm down from the top of the dividing line (with considerable image jump). It was originally made in plus-cylinder form then was manufactured in minus-cylinder form. Designed as compromise general-purpose occupational lenses, Ultex E bifocals were phased out by manufacturers in the United States but still prescribed in some foreign countries. The shape/size is used for some high-add designs for the low-vision patient in the United States.

Ultex A (38mm × 19mm)

The Ultex A is a semicircular segment measuring 38mm across at its widest point, with an optical center 19mm below the dividing line (Figure 3.13). The manufacturing process is like that of the Ultex E. When the bevel allowance is made, the maximum segment height is 18mm or 18.5mm. If a higher segment is needed, the practitioner specifies Ultex AA (sometimes called Ultex AL; Figure 3.14). The laboratory then utilizes one factory blank to obtain a single finished lens. Designed as a vocational bifocal, the style was unique at its conception, offering an exceptionally large reading area. Today the wide range of large segments having little or no image jump has reduced considerably the use of the Ultex A in the United States. Originally manufactured in plus-cylinder form only, it is now available in a minus-cylinder design.

Note: When the term *Ultex* is used without other identification, laboratories and practitioners are referring to the Ultex A-type design.

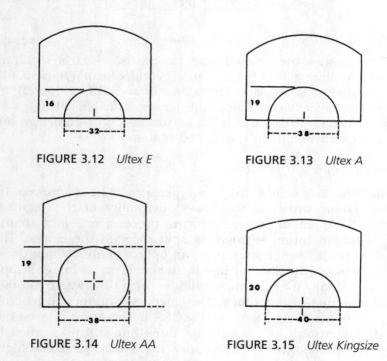

FIGURE 3.12   *Ultex E*   FIGURE 3.13   *Ultex A*

FIGURE 3.14   *Ultex AA*   FIGURE 3.15   *Ultex Kingsize*

Ultex Kingsize (40mm × 20mm)

The Ultex Kingsize was a 40mm semicircular occupational bifocal, plus-cylinder lens manufactured in the same manner as the Ultex A and Ultex E (Figure 3.15). The factory blank results in two finished lenses, each having an optical center 20mm below the dividing line. This bifocal was then made in a minus-cylinder design, but it is rarely prescribed in the United States because of the large amount of image jump.

Rede-Rite (Minus Add) Bifocal (38mm × 19mm)

The Rede-Rite looks like an inverted Ultex A bifocal with the semicircular segment in the upper portion of the lens (Figure 3.16). Manufacturers identify it as a reading bifocal with a distance window. It was one of the original minus-add bifocals, but inverted segments are rarely worn today because patients prefer large-segment, occupational bifocals. The Rede-Rite is still listed in some catalogues as currently available.

High-Lite B Style (22mm Round)

This 22mm round bifocal is fashioned from one piece of high-index 1.7 glass, so the curves are flatter and the lens considerably thinner than a comparable crown glass correction (Figure 3.17). High-Lite B style was designed specifically as a cosmetic lens for patients needing −6.00D or more in the distance correction. However, because high-index is "heavy" glass and exhibits considerable chromatic aberration, this lens was rarely prescribed and may no longer be available.

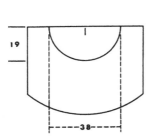

FIGURE 3.16 *Rede-Rite*

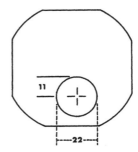

FIGURE 3.17 *High-Lite B style*

High-Lite A Style (38mm × 19mm)

The High-Lite A style is an occupational, one-piece bifocal, index 1.7, designed as a cosmetically acceptable lens for high myopes (Figure 3.18). The weight of the lens, the position of the optical center, 19mm below the dividing line, and chromatic aberration severely limit its use. It may no longer be available.

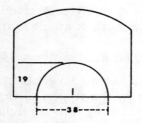

FIGURE 3.18   *High-Lite A style*

POSITIONING THE BIFOCAL FOR CONVENTIONAL WEAR: FIRST-TIME WEARER

For patients wearing bifocals for the first time, it is customary to place the segment line of straight-top (flat-top) and curve-top general-purpose bifocals 1mm beneath the lower lid. Most first-time wearers find this positioning satisfactory. When a patient has worn bifocals for a period of time, a slightly higher or lower position may be requested, and the segment height altered accordingly.

The round-top segment is placed a millimeter or so higher (at the lower lid) than the straight-segment designs because patients need to tilt the neck farther back to utilize the maximum-width near area (through the optical center). In addition, the dividing line is not prominent and the higher positioning is not likely to be an annoyance.

PROCEDURE FOR MEASUREMENT OF BIFOCAL HEIGHT

To measure the segment top to the lower edge of the lens, the following seven steps should be performed *in the order given:*

1. Place the selected frame on the patient's face.
2. Hold the frame in the position it will occupy when the final fitting takes place.
3. With the examiner's eyes and the patient's eyes *on the same level,* a plastic ophthalmic ruler is placed vertically over the rims (or the lens, if it is a rimless mounting) with the zero point positioned as though it were the top of the bifocal.
4. Note the reading. If the frame shape is an aviator-type or cut off nasally, the lens must be mentally blocked

into a box shape and the reading estimated to the lower lens edge (Figure 3.19).

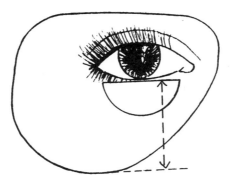

FIGURE 3.19

5. If the frame sample is the correct size and it is a wire, rimless, combination, or combination-type mounting, order the observed reading. For plastic designs, add 0.5mm for light-weight and medium-weight frames and 1mm for heavy-weight or extra-heavy-weight frames. This allows for the lens bevel that fits into the groove of the rims.

6. If the sample eyesize varies from the finished eyewear, the allowance is 1mm for each 2mm difference. For example, a 52mm eyesize frame is used to determine the bifocal height, but a 54mm eyesize is ordered. The finished lens will be 1mm wider all around, so another 1mm is added to the measurement.

7. If the patient has a hyper eye, each segment height is measured separately. Only one-half the allowance is made, however, because the difference is partially compensated for by the frame adjustment on the face.

Example:

The right segment measures 18mm high, the left measures 20mm high. Order 18.5mm for the right lens and 19.5mm for the left. The patient with a hyper eye finds the eyewear more comfortable when angled during the final fitting in the direction of the higher eye.

There are certain conditions requiring bifocal positionings other than those described above. If the correction is used primarily for close work and is rarely worn for distance viewing, segments set 2mm or 3mm above the lower lid allow for more comfortable head/neck posture. On the other hand, patients who wear bifocals in a sunglass correction often request slightly lower segments so that the division between far and near will not interfere with operating a motor vehicle.

Literature sometimes suggests that bifocals be set low when dispensed to physically challenged people, but these patients should not be given bifocal lenses (or any multifocal lens). Unsure of their footing when looking through the adds, they can stumble and fall. This is a serious consideration, particularly with elderly patients who have great difficulty recovering from injuries. If in doubt, it is always best to recommend two pairs: one for distance and the other for near viewing.

SEGMENT HEIGHT FOR A PREVIOUS BIFOCAL WEARER

If a patient has been wearing a bifocal correction and the case history indicates satisfaction, the new segments should occupy the same position on the face. With the patient wearing the previous correction, note the position of the segments in relation to the lower lid. (The examiner and the patient must be on the *same eye level.*) With the new frame in position, place the zero point of the ruler where the top of the bifocal will be placed. Proceed as previously outlined.

Note: It is critical that optically designed plastic rulers or segment measures be used. Inexpensive flexible rulers may give a false reading; metal rulers have been known to slip and injure the patient's face.

Chapter 4

GLASS TRIFOCAL
DESIGNS

INTRODUCTION

While bifocals fulfill a need for the beginning presbyope by providing clear vision at distance and near, as the patient grows older, the accommodative mechanism becomes less flexible. Eventually a point is reached when the bifocal segment does not provide an adequate range for both near and intermediate clear vision, usually noticed when the near add reaches a power of +1.75D. Clear vision at all distances can be restored by the addition of an intermediate add of less plus power than the near segment. This, then, is the advantage and the reason for the trifocal design. As the name implies, the trifocal lens has three foci: a distance correction, an intermediate power, and a near add.

Most modern trifocals are manufactured with the power of the intermediate segment 50% that of the near add. For most patients, this 50% intermediate provides an excellent range of clear vision. In the few cases in which this power is inadequate, the correct prescription is easily determined by a trial frame refraction. The lens can be then ordered in a design that fulfills the patient's visual requirements.

It is rarely necessary or advisable to start a beginning multifocal wearer with a trifocal correction. Bifocals are almost always adequate for first-time multifocal wearers because the add is usually relatively low in power. Furthermore, bifocals afford the patient an easier way of adjusting to the dividing line (single instead of double). In addition, optical drawbacks such as object displacement, image jump, and limitations of the near field are easier to overcome when only one segment is involved.

When the necessary add becomes +1.75D or more, it is good to consider prescribing a trifocal lens. Some patients do not require clear vision at intermediate distances and are not inconvenienced when wearing bifocals. In many cases, however, modern needs necessitate clear vision at all distances. Many patients (e.g., homemakers involved in numerous intermediate tasks such as ironing, washing, cooking, and bedmaking) are not aware of the advantages of a trifocal lens and need to have them brought to their attention. Once patients have worn trifocals, they find it difficult to be satisfied with the limitations of a bifocal design.

In the fitting of trifocal lenses, it is usually best to position the upper line of the intermediate segment 1mm below the pupil in normal daytime illumination (the procedure is the same as that outlined for bifocal fitting in Chapter 3, "Prescribing Modern Glass Bifocal Designs"). Most of the problems encountered in trifocal fitting stem from positioning the intermediate segment too high, resulting in a dividing line that is difficult to ignore when using the lenses for distance viewing.

To allow for an adequate near add, the trifocal segment for conventional wear should be at least 20mm high, including the intermediate area. This height is sometimes difficult to obtain when narrow-lens/large-difference frames are prescribed. However, with the current variety of frame designs available, it is always possible to find a cosmetically pleasing style into which this segment height can be fit (occupational trifocals must be set higher than 20mm for an adequate near area. An in-depth case history will determine the patient's needs).

CONSTRUCTION OF FUSED TRIFOCALS

Trifocals are manufactured in the same basic designs as bifocals. Like the bifocal, the fused form consists of a major lens blank fashioned of crown glass and segments constructed of a barium-flint combination. The countersink curve in the major blank is shaped to fit both the intermediate and near buttons. Obviously, to obtain the proper powers, the index of the near button is higher than that of the intermediate. All fused trifocals manufactured in the United States are made in minus-cylinder form with the segments on the outside surface of the lens.

For better understanding of fused bifocal designs, some of the mathematical computations involved in their manufacture are discussed in Chapter 2, "Introduction to Bifocal Lenses." Basically, the same principles are applicable to the manufacture of fused trifocal designs, the only difference being that two segment powers are involved: the intermediate add and the near add. The following additional problems relating exclusively to trifocals are given for the interested scholar (the term *Kryptok factor* remains by common usage).

PROBLEM:

A trifocal lens has a distance power of +3.00D with a near add of +3.00D and a 50% intermediate power. The index of the distance portion is 1.5; the power of the countersink curve is −4.00D; the power of the inside curve is −6.00D. Find the following:
(a) the index of the intermediate segment
(b) the index of the near segment

PROCEDURE FOR (A):

1. Determine the Kryptok factor (remains by common usage) for the intermediate.

$$K_f = \frac{F_{front} - F_{cc}}{F_{add \text{ (intermediate portion)}}}$$

$$= \frac{+9.00 - (-4.00)}{+1.50}$$

$$= 8.67$$

2. Use the Kryptok factor to determine the index of the intermediate.

$$\text{Since } K_f = \frac{n_d - 1}{n_n - n_d}$$

$$n_n = \frac{(n_d - 1) + K_f n_d}{K_f}$$

$$= \frac{(1.5 - 1) + (8.67)(1.5)}{8.67}$$

$$= 1.56$$

SOLUTION TO (a):

Index of the intermediate = 1.56

PROCEDURE FOR (b):

1.   Determine the Kryptok factor (remains by common usage) for the near portion.

$$K_f = \frac{K_{front} - F_{cc}}{F_{add}}$$

$$= \frac{+9.00 - (-4.00)}{+3.00}$$

$$= 4.33$$

2.   Use the Kryptok factor to determine the index of the near portion.

$$n_n = \frac{(n_d - 1) + K_f n_d}{K_f}$$

$$= \frac{(1.5 - 1) + (4.33)(1.5)}{4.33}$$

$$= 1.62$$

SOLUTION TO (b):

Index of the near portion = 1.62

PROBLEM:

A straight-top 7-25 (also called flat top 7-25) fused trifocal with a distance prescription of $-2.00 - .50 \times 90$ has a near add of +2.75D and a 50% intermediate. The power of the countersink curve is $-3.00D$ and of the back surface is $-8.00D$. The distance index is 1.523. Find the following:
(a) the index of the intermediate segment
(b) the index of the near segment

PROCEDURE FOR (a):

1. Determine the Kryptok factor for the intermediate.

$$K_f = \frac{F_{front} - F_{cc}}{F_{add}}$$

$$= \frac{+6.00 - (-3.00)}{+1.37}$$

$$= 6.569$$

2. Determine the index of the intermediate using the Kryptok factor.

$$n_n = \frac{(n_d - 1) + K_f n_d}{K_f}$$

$$= \frac{(1.523 - 1) + (6.569)(1.523)}{6.569}$$

$$= 1.60$$

SOLUTION TO (a):

Index of the intermediate segment $= 1.60$

PROCEDURE FOR (b):

1. Determine the Kryptok factor (by common usage) for the near portion.

$$K_f = \frac{K_{front} - F_{cc}}{F_{add}}$$

$$= \frac{+6.00 - (-3.00)}{+2.75}$$

$$= 3.273$$

2. Determine the index of the near portion using the Kryptok factor.

$$n_n = \frac{(n_d - 1) + K_f n_d}{K_f}$$

$$= \frac{(1.523 - 1) + (3.273)(1.523)}{3.273}$$

$$= 1.68$$

SOLUTION TO **(b)**:

Index of the near segment = 1.68

FUSED TRIFOCAL DESIGNS

Flat-top (Also Called Straight-top) Fused Trifocals

The straight-top (flat-top) fused trifocal was introduced by Univis Lens Co. The design features two straight dividing lines, the upper separating the distance from the intermediate segment and the lower separating the intermediate segment from the near. In the standard designs, the lower segment is curved in a half-round pattern. In most catalogues, this lens is designated by two numbers, the first giving the height of the intermediate segment and the second, the maximum width of the near add.

Example:

Flat-top (straight-top) 7-25 (sometimes written FT7/25 or 7 × 25) trifocal means the intermediate height is 7mm and the maximum width of the near segment is 25mm. (One catalogue lists the design as 7 TRI 25, meaning 7mm high intermediate and 25mm at the widest near area.)

Most glass trifocals are manufactured with the intermediate segment equal to one-half the power of the near. Therefore, if the near add is +2.50D, the intermediate is +1.25D. The few designs having available varying powers will be noted when explaining the lens. The 50% intermediate is automatically supplied by the local laboratory unless otherwise specified.

The straight-top designs (also called flat top) are the most widely prescribed trifocals in the United States in CR 39, polycarbonates, and glass. Most manufacturers place the near optical center 3mm below the division separating intermediate from near.

Flat-top (Straight-top) 6-22mm, 6-25mm, and 7-23mm

These trifocals were among the first general-purpose, flat-top designs. They are rarely prescribed today because by modern standards the segment areas are limiting in size. (ST6-22 is shown in Figure 4.1.)

Flat-top 7-25
(Also Listed in Catalogues as Straight-top 7 × 25 or 7 TRI 25)

The ST7-25mm is a widely prescribed trifocal. Its size makes it a good general-purpose lens (Figure 4.2), although practitioners tend to prefer the FT 7-28. On special order, depending on the power, the intermediate segment is available with an add that is 40%, 60%, or 70% of the near, in addition to the standard 50%.

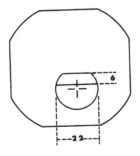

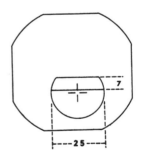

FIGURE 4.1 *Flat-top 6-22*   **FIGURE 4.2** *Flat-top 7-25*

Flat-top 7-28 (Also Straight-top 7 × 28 or 7 TRI 28)

Although the ST7-28 was originally designed as an occupational trifocal, its comfortable reading area has made it a lens of popular choice for the patient desiring a compromise general-purpose, large-segment multifocal (Figure 4.3). Aside from the standard 50%, it can be specially ordered with an intermediate power that is 40% or 60% of the near add. Its popularity makes it easily available in a number of standard colors: Photogray

Extra; Photobrown Extra; pink 1 and 2; gray 1, 2, and 3; green 1, 2, and 3. Other colors can be obtained by coating the lens.

Flat-top 7-35 (Also Called Straight-top 7 × 35 or 7 TRI 35)

The ST7-35 is a vocational "large-segment" trifocal (Figure 4.4). Because of the size of the segments, the dividing lines are relatively prominent. However, if cosmetic appearance is not a problem, this lens supplies an excellent near field for the patient who needs it. The add is also large enough to create prism at the near point by decentration. In these cases, the lens is worn as a general-purpose trifocal, and although the dividing lines are prominent, this form of correction is cosmetically superior to having the prism ground into the segment. (Prism segments are available in bifocal form only. This also is a limitation.) This lens is available in Photogray Extra; Photobrown Extra; pink 1 and 2; gray 1, 2, and 3; green 1, 2, and 3. As with all glass lenses, color coatings in any desired shade can be ordered.

Flat-top 8-25 (Also Called Straight-top 8 × 25 and 8 TRI 25)

This trifocal, which has an 8mm intermediate height, is rarely prescribed (practitioners and patients tend to prefer the 7 × 25 as a general-purpose trifocal). It is available in only a few standard tints and current catalogues should be consulted.

Flat-top 8-28

Like the flat top 8-25, this is a rarely prescribed lens, and standard tints are limited. The local laboratory can be queried for specifics.

Flat-top 10-25, Flat-top 10-28

Both the flat top 10-25 and the flat top 10-28 are designed for patients needing a large intermediate segment. However, they are rarely prescribed because the flat-top 10-35, described below, more adequately fulfills the needs of these patients (can be listed as 10 TRI 25 and 10 TRI 28).

Flat-top 10-35 (Also Called Straight-top 10 × 35, 10 TRI 35)

This trifocal is designed for patients needing large intermediate and near segments (Figure 4.5). It is meant as an occupational trifocal and serves best when the dividing line separating the intermediate from the distance correction is set into the pupil area. Otherwise, the patient has to maintain an uncomfortable head-back position to utilize the near segment efficiently.

Note: Vision-Ease Lens specializes in unusual-size, custom straight-top glass trifocals. If a special combination of intermediate and near segments is desired, availability can be ascertained by querying the local laboratory.

UNUSUAL STRAIGHT-TOP GLASS TRIFOCAL DESIGNS

R-Style Trifocal (6-22mm) (Also Called Ribbon Trifocal)

This trifocal features an R-style bifocal segment for the near area; the upper and lower divisions are straight lines (Figure 4.6). It is listed as available but it is rarely, if ever, prescribed. In almost every case, conventional general-purpose, straight-top trifocals better serve the patient's needs in design and size.

Univis Ultra CV (Glass; Discontinued)

This trifocal, originally manufactured by Univis is no longer available. It featured a 20mm D-shaped near add in a 30mm D-shaped intermediate area (Figure 4.7). Patients wearing the design need to be given another trifocal style.

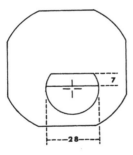

FIGURE 4.3   *Flat-top 7-28*

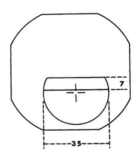

FIGURE 4.4   *Flat-top 7-35*

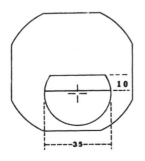

FIGURE 4.5   *Flat-top 10-35*

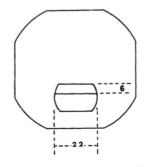

FIGURE 4.6   *R-style 6-22*

CURVED-TOP FUSED TRIFOCAL

Curved-top Trifocal

This design, introduced by American Optical Corp., features an intermediate segment that combines curved upper and lower borders with sharp corners. The lower-segment area has the same appearance as the Sovereign bifocal. The original lens incorporated a 25mm near segment with a 7mm intermediate (Figure 4.8). This trifocal is now available with a 24mm-wide near segment (instead of 25mm) but is rarely prescribed.

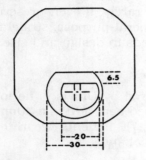

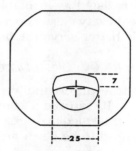

FIGURE 4.7   *Ultra CV (glass)*
(discontinued)

FIGURE 4.8   *Curved-top trifocal*

Panoptik Trifocal (Discontinued)

The Panoptik trifocal, created by Bausch & Lomb, combined a 7mm intermediate segment with a 25mm near add (Figure 4.9). It featured an intermediate segment having a slightly curved top with rounded corners; the near add was D-shaped, and the two areas were separated by a straight dividing line. The lens featured a 50% intermediate when last manufactured, although in past years the intermediate power varied according to the power of the add (known as the *Functional Panoptik*). The lens style is no longer available. It is unlikely that patients are still wearing the design, but if so, they need to be prescribed a suitable flat-top trifocal.

ONE-PIECE GLASS TRIFOCALS

One-piece trifocal construction is basically similar to that of the one-piece bifocal. However, instead of two curvatures on the spherical surface of the lens, the needed power for intermediate and near add is obtained by three changes in curvature.

ONE-PIECE TRIFOCAL DESIGNS

Executive (Straight-across Trifocal)

This one-piece trifocal, originally distributed by American Optical Corp. under the trade name Executive trifocal, features two straight dividing lines extending across the entire lens. The intermediate area is 7mm high and has a power that is 50% of the near add (Figure 4.10). It is an excellent occupational design because the size supplies the widest segment field of any conventional trifocal. The near optical center is placed on the line dividing the intermediate from the near add. The positioning of the optical center cancels all image jump when fixation is altered from one segment area to another. However, there are several disadvantages. The segments, located on the nonocular surface, have protruding shelves that tend to chip unless the patient exercises care in handling the glasses. The shelves are extremely prominent, and from a cosmetic viewpoint, this trifocal is less desirable than other designs. It is best to show the patient a sample lens before ordering. Appearance may be a significant factor to consider. This trifocal is not desirable as a general-purpose lens. The distance area is too limiting, especially when the lens is worn while operating a motor vehicle.

Ultex T (Discontinued)

The Ultex T featured a near add, 19mm round surrounded by a circular band, 6mm wide (Figure 4.11). Never a popular design, it has been discontinued for at least a decade. If a patient is still wearing this lens, another style must be prescribed.

Ultex X

This lens is still listed in catalogues, but availability may be a problem. The design was created by Continental Optical Co. and features a semicircular near segment measuring 32mm wide on the factory blank (Figure 4.12). The 8mm intermediate circular band has a power 50% that of the near, although at one time it varied according to the add. Considerable image jump created by the position of the near optical center (16mm below the lower dividing line) makes it undesirable in view of the superior optics of more recent trifocal designs.

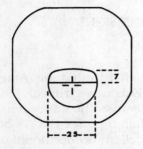

FIGURE 4.9   Panoptik trifocal (discontinued)

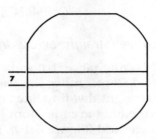

FIGURE 4.10   Straight-across trifocal

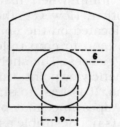

FIGURE 4.11   Ultex T (discontinued)

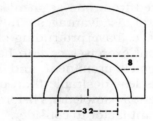

FIGURE 4.12   Ultex X

CONCLUSION

Glass lenses in all designs occupy only about 30% of the lens market. Whenever possible, it is best to prescribe a polycarbonate plastic trifocal design (see Chapter 7, "Plastic Ophthalmic Lenses"). Glass trifocal lenses have a wider range of designs/prescriptions, but the availability of plastic multifocals is rapidly expanding. The local laboratory should be queried frequently for updates.

PRESCRIBING "INVISIBLE" MULTIFOCALS

INTRODUCTION

The association of bifocals with visual problems of middle age brought about attempts to design lenses that would be difficult to identify cosmetically as multifocals. This was inevitable. There are patients for whom the psychological, social, and occupational advantages of a youthful appearance are of prime importance.

A great number of "invisible" multifocals are available; all look like single-vision lenses when the patient is viewed full face. However, the power changes separating the near and/or intermediate areas sometimes are obvious when the wearer's head is tilted. Without exception, the major optical problem is the presence of unwanted cylinder, which causes distorted vision when the patient looks through certain sections of the lens.

The original designs, and still available, are bifocals that have an optically sound distance portion and an accurate near correction, the latter surrounded by a blur circle. For the most part, however, patients desiring a multifocal without lines are prescribed progressive addition-type lenses (PALs). The distance prescription is followed by power increases in a series of adds until a full near correction is reached. All such lenses have certain peripheral areas that exhibit distortion.

The earlier American-distributed variable power lens designs were the Omnifocal introduced by Univis about four decades ago, the Progressor distributed by Titmus Optical in the late 1960s, and the Varilux 1 of the same era. All have been replaced by vastly improved designs. PALs are today manufactured and/or distributed by all major lens companies. Some of the designs are so similar that they could be interchangeable. Specifics of certain PALs are described in this chapter. These are limited primarily to widely advertised designs since basically all others are versions of these lenses. Studying the literature distributed to the eyecare professional with each lens as it is released is critical to understanding its optical design.

SEAMLESS (BLENDED) BIFOCALS

Younger Seamless Bifocal

While PALs are much more in use than the seamless lens, an explanation of the Younger seamless bifocal is first in order because it was the original no-line multifocal.

Younger Optics introduced the first seamless bifocal in 1954 and is still the world's largest manufacturer. *Seamless* is a Younger Optics–copyrighted trade name; other manufacturers refer to the style as *blended bifocals*. The dividing line that exists in conventional round-top bifocals is polished out, resulting in a barely perceptible blur circle. The seamless lens is a one-piece, minus-cylinder design and is currently available in CR 39 plastic and Photogray Extra glass.

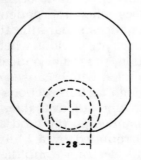

FIGURE 5.1   *Younger Seamless bifocal—CR 39*

The CR 39 plastic design (Figure 5.1) is made with a 28mm-across full reading field. The width of the distorted area surrounding this field is about 3mm. Like all CR 39 plastic, the lens can be tinted any desired color. The Photogray Extra, designed as an indoor-outdoor seamless bifocal, is available with a 22mm-wide near field. The circling distorted area is about 3mm, varying slightly depending on the prescription. The lower adds result in more flare-out, while the transition in the higher adds is better controlled. (The older 18mm and 20mm segment sizes were discontinued decades ago. The high-index glass, 1.7, has also been discontinued. It felt heavy on the face and, like all high-index glass lenses, exhibited pronounced color aberration.)

The Seamless bifocal is called the *blended lens* by other manufacturers and available with a 25mm useable near area. The CR 39, 25mm segment is manufactured by Phillips Lens Co. under the trade name Ultimate. Signet Armorlite distributes a comparable lens, as does the Vision-Ease Lens Co.

The major disadvantage of Seamless blended bifocals is the distortion characteristic of the blur circle. When a spherical distance correction is involved, a cylinder power is induced that is uncontrollable in both amount and axis. If the correction is a sphero-cylinder, the blur area introduces a new cylinder power at an uncontrollable axis.

Younger Optics states that the Seamless (blended) lens is generally worn with satisfaction when it is the patient's first bifocal (a lower add means less distortion). Experience has shown that the patient must also be cosmetically motivated. Learning to ignore the distorted areas can be a problem. However, there are patients concerned enough with cosmesis they will wear this design particularly for social activities.

For prolonged periods of comfortable near work, it is probably best to also prescribe a separate pair of reading glasses or a flat-top 28mm bifocal. This insures that the patient has eyewear that fits most visual needs.

Fitting Seamless (Blended) Bifocals

Unlike PALs, blended bifocals are easy to fit. There is the suggestion that it is best to measure the bifocal height as though the blended lens were a round-top bifocal, usually to the top of the lower lid, and then adding 1mm (see Chapter 3, "Prescribing Modern Glass Bifocal Designs" for the actual technique). However, ordering the blur area to start about 3mm above the lower lid margin usually better serves the patient as it allows for a more normal head/neck position for close viewing. Younger Optics, the original manufacturer, suggests that the measurement be even higher, as though it were a trifocal. That is a logical recommendation.

There may be a problem communicating with the laboratory regarding segment height. The practitioner *must be specific* when ordering. If the top of the blur area is to be 1mm below the pupil margin in normal illumination (as in a trifocal), this must be stated under "Special Instructions." Left on their own, most technicians set the blur circle 0.5mm above and 0.5mm below the height given. For instance, the ordered height is 22mm; the blur area is 3mm wide, so 1.5mm blur is above 22mm (at 23.5mm) and 1.5mm is below. The patient, therefore, has a usable near field that is 20.5mm high.

While an accurate P.D. is important, a monocular P.D. is not necessary. (A monocular P.D. is critical when measuring for a PAL.)

PROGRESSIVE ADDITION LENSES

Progressive addition lenses have made remarkable strides within the optical industry. All designs feature adds in a normal progression for clear vision as the patient looks down. However, all have some type of distortion in the periphery of the lens surrounding the add powers. This distortion is usually identified as *hard* for pronounced peripheral distortion and *soft* for lenses having less distortion.

The hard designs have a wider true power area for the total near add but may be less tolerable to the patient because of the "swimming" effect when walking. The hard design is almost always recommended for prolonged near tasks (e.g., working at a computer) because of the wider true power. The softer designs narrow the zone of clear vision but because the distortion is less pronounced may be easier to wear.

Manufacturers of the newer PALs sometimes hesitate to use the terms *hard* or *soft* because they incorporate a balance between the two and refer to the lens as *multi-design*, explaining that it combines the best of spherical and aspheric designs.

The most widely recognized PAL because of extensive advertising on television is the Varilux Comfort (Essilor of America) available in a wide variety of lens materials. Before this lens is described, a background of the original Varilux as well as other original designs is in order. They laid the basic principles for the PALs prescribed today.

HISTORICAL PROSPECTIVE

Original Varilux (Multi-Optics)

The first PAL to have a real impact on the multifocal field was the Varilux 1, distributed in the late 1950s and early 1960s. The first steps toward developing this multifocal without visible dividing lines and featuring a gradual increase in plus add powers were taken in the early 1950s by Société des Lundtiers of Paris, France. In 1959, marketing was started. In 1975 another version, referred to as Varilux 2, was manufactured by Essex Silor and distributed by Essilor International of France. When it was made available in the United States by Multi-Optics, a division of Essilor, it was simply called Varilux. (The current Varilux Comfort is a registered trademark of Essilor of America.)

The Varilux 1 and Varilux 2 featured three major optical zones. The upper portion of the lens contained the distance prescription; the intermediate zone proceeded from zero add and gradually increased in power until the near correction was reached. The remainder of the clear optical zone consisted of the full near power. Vision was allowed to pass from distance to near in a gradual, smooth manner. The lenses were a one-piece type of construction with the changes in curvature placed on the front surface by the factory; the concave side was spherical, cylindrical, prismatic, or any combination of these powers, depending on the prescription, and ground by the local laboratory. Basically, the concept of current PALs still follows this pattern.

Fitting procedure for the Varilux was the same as it is today for all PALs. Since the intermediate and near decentrations are predetermined, conventional multifocal segment heights must be replaced by two measurements that allow the lenses to align horizontally and vertically. The first of these is a monocular P.D. *Accuracy is critical* so a pupillometer must be used to eliminate the margin of error normally attributed to parallax. Equally as important is the distance from the reference point on the pupil (usually the center of the pupil) to the lower edge of the lens. This measurement is taken with the *correct frame style and size in place* while the patient, fixating on a distance object, assumes natural head and eye posture. Each eye *must be measured separately* because facial asymmetry may be present. It is critical that the distorted areas be reached simultaneously when the patient looks down. When the lens is fit according to these specifications, the progressive and full add areas will assume proper positioning.

For the original Varilux, an adequate-size near correction involved a measurement from the center of the pupil to the lower lens edge of at least 22mm. This still holds for most PALs but there is more leeway in some of today's designs. These are discussed later in this chapter. The Varilux 1 exhibited an optically perfect distance portion (Figure 5.2). The distorted areas characteristic of all PALs were concentrated in the periphery surrounding the intermediate and near corrections. Today that would be called a hard design.

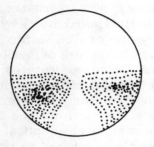

FIGURE 5.2   *Original Varilux 1*

The later Varilux 2 design spread out the distortion to reduce the rocking motion induced by uncontrollable cylindrical power in amount and axis. There was some aberration in certain peripheral portions of the distance, as well as a size reduction in the optically correct near zone (Figure 5.3). That would be called a soft design today.

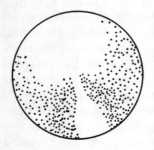

FIGURE 5.3   *Original Varilux 2*

HISTORICAL PROSPECTIVE (CONTINUED)

Ultravue Progressive Power Lenses
(American Optical; Discontinued)

This lens is important historically because the reference terms of the Ultravue Progressive Power lenses became part of the terminology of PALs. The series of add powers through which the eye travels from distance to near is called the *progressive corridor.* The term *optically pure* was coined to designate the areas of the prescribed correction to differentiate them from the distorted sections common to all PALs.

In the Ultravue, there was a relatively wide optically pure near portion, resulting in intense peripheral distortion surrounding the add powers. Such patterns are now identified as a hard design (Figure 5.4).

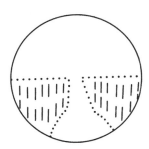

FIGURE 5.4   *Ultravue (discontinued)*

This lens is also important historically because in an era in which most lenses were fashioned of glass, the Ultravue was made only in hard-resin CR 39 plastic identified as Aolite Ultravue. It also came in two sizes: Ultravue 25 (width of near area); later an Ultravue 28 was added. This too was unusual because PALs tended to be identified with one set of dimensions, although there are some variations in all PALs depending on the prescription. It was also important to note that American Optical introduced the Grolman Fitting System recommended for "absolute accuracy" in fitting the Ultravue, while, in truth, following the instructions by any manufacturer will give the necessary information.

HISTORICAL PROSPECTIVE (CONTINUED)

Younger 10/30 Consecutive Power Lenses and Younger CPS Progressives (Younger Optics; Both Discontinued)

Although these lenses are no longer manufactured (Younger Optics makes the Image PAL only), they were important in their day. The first number of the Younger 10/30 represented the 10mm that was both the length of the transition zone and its width; the number 30 identified the effective diameter of the near area. The Younger CPS (consecutive power parabolic sphere) was one of the first to feature curves that attempted to minimize peripheral distortion.

CURRENT PAL DESIGNS

Currently available PALs are described here, but not all are mentioned nor are they in any special order. Those widely advertised to the eyecare professions and/or to the public are included. In truth, specific designs by various distributors are released with such regularity that the eyecare professional must study the literature distributed with each PAL. With an understanding the basic optics/use as described in this chapter, it is then simple to know which designs to recommend and/or prescribe.

Varilux Comfort (Essilor of America)

Today's Varilux Comfort lens is the most widely advertised PAL in history. Television coverage is intense, appearing daily on a great number of network and cable stations throughout the United States. Publications slanted toward mature persons also feature extensive advertising campaigns spotlighting the Varilux Comfort lens.

The distance area of this lens is relatively free of distortion—85% of the full add is reached 12mm below the fitting cross. The full add is then achieved at 18mm below the fitting cross. It is described as a soft design, meaning that the distorted areas are spread out and less likely to cause major problems. Like all soft designs, there is less area for the full add. The manufacturer states that the exact measurements for the clear zones depend upon the prescription.

To fill a wide range of needs, the Varilux Comfort is advertised as offering more premium material choices than any other PAL.

In addition to polycarbonate (called Airwear) choices are Orma CR 39 hard resin as well as a special CR 39 called UVX, which offers complete protection against ultraviolet radiations. There is also Ormex (1.55 high-index plastic), Thin and Lite (1.60 high-index plastic), clear crown glass, Photogray Extra and Photobrown Extra. Polarized sunlenses are available, as are Transitions Gray and Transitions Brown absorptive designs. The Transitions Gray becomes virtually clear indoors. The Transition XTRActive is a darker gray tint outdoors and remains a light gray indoors. The Ormex 1.55 high-index Transitions Gray and Brown are the thinnest, lightest lens material in a photochromic lens. (Further details are in Chapter 9, "Prescribing Absorptive Lenses.")

Essilor Natural (Essilor of America)

For patients needing a fuller near area of a useable prescription than with the Varilux Comfort, Essilor offers the Essilor Natural with a wider near and intermediate field. Essilor advertises the lens as the best of both hard and soft PALs with distortion softened in the periphery (could be identified as a multi-design). Eighty-five percent of the full add is 14mm below the fitting cross. The full add power is reached 18mm below the fitting cross. It is available in a number of lens materials, including polycarbonates; 1.5 Ormex high-index plastic; Ormex Transitions Gray; Index 1.5; and Transitions Gray, Transitions Brown, and Transitions XTRActive.

Silor-Adaptor and Silor-Nuline (Essilor of America)

To further enable prescribing for patients needing a fuller clear area for near than obtainable with the Varilux Comfort or Essilor Natural, Essilor offers the Silor-Adaptor (harder than the two above-mentioned designs) and the Silor-Nuline, the hardest of the four (most peripheral distortion). The maximum width of the total near power is 18mm below the fitting cross. Prescribing either of these two lenses depends on the patient's case history and the expertise of the eyecare practitioner, who must take into consideration the intense peripheral distortion.

Note: Essilor makes a lens that is only partially a progressive addition design. It is called Varilux Overview. The lower part of the lens is a normal Varilux progressive addition. The upper area carries a 41mm bifocal shaped like a half-moon. The distance between the central fitting cross and the segment edge is 9mm. The upper add power is always 0.50D less than the full add (e.g., for a +2.00D maximum near, the add at the top is +1.50D). The manufacturer recommends the Varilux Overview for technicians, mechanics, painters, and librarians. It is discussed also in Chapter 6, "Prescribing Double-segment and Quadrifocal Lenses."

Technica (American Optical)

The Technica by American Optical is advertised as a vision correction for computer use. It has wide intermediate useable areas and a wide near area. Distortion therefore is concentrated in the periphery (a hard progressive addition design). The Technica is meant for the patient using the lens while sitting down as there is a considerable "swimming" effect if worn when walking. The Technica is available in plastic CR 39. The manufacturer recommends a light pink or a light gray tint be incorporated because computer users often become light sensitive, particularly if there is overhead fluorescent lighting. Antireflection coatings could also be applied to reduce ghost images, but it must be remembered that they will not eliminate glare from the screen.

Compact Progressive (American Optical)

In 1999, American Optical Lens Company introduced the Compact PAL designed for small/narrowed frames (similar to Image, Figure 5.5). It is identified as multi-design (neither hard nor soft). Manufactured in CR 39 plastic, it needs only a minimum frame depth of 17mm for a full-power reading area (rather than the 22mm or 23mm for most PALs). This is accomplished by limiting the corridor length to 13mm, which is about 4mm less than average (corridor length determines size of reading area). American Optical suggests that there is no need to increase the add by 0.25D, as is sometimes recommended with PALs. The manufacturer suggests that the A Perma Cote Advanced Hard Coating be applied to enhance the scratch resistance of the CR 39 plastic.

The Compact Progressive lens has not been worn long enough to judge patient reaction, but it is logical to assume that for dress wear, patients will enjoy this cosmetically pleasing lens. It is compatible with many of the newer frame designs that are currently in fashion. As is recommended with other PALs, additional eyewear with corrections free of distortion are highly recommended for prolonged comfortable wear.

TruVision Progressive (American Optical)

TruVision was one of the original hard PALs. There is some peripheral distortion above the 0° to 180° line (similar to original Varilux). The corridor is about 16mm in length, and the near useable area is a circle about 24mm wide surrounded by intense distortion. The deeper corridor allows for more natural use of the intermediate add powers but does mean there is more neck/head tilt to reach the widest area of the near correction. It is currently available in CR 39 plastic, crown glass, and some photochromic glass designs.

Omni (American Optical)

American Optical makes a soft design called Omni. It is available in polycarbonate, CR 39 plastic, clear crown glass, and some photochromic glass designs. As in all soft designs, the distortion surrounding the intermediate and near areas is spread out so it is easier for the patient to adjust to wearing the lens. However, characteristic of all soft designs, the result is a smaller near field than with a hard progressive lens.

Image (Younger Optics)

The Image is designed to be compatible with narrowed-vertical-dimension frames. From the fitting cross to the bottom of the lens, the measurement can be as small as 18mm (instead of the 22mm recommended for most PALs). The Image PAL is relatively free of distortion in the distance area. Distortion surrounding the intermediate and near areas has been kept to a minimum. Younger describes the lens as an aspheric design, but the description could also identify it as a soft progressive or possibly a multi-design lens (Figure 5.5).

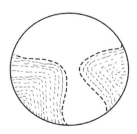

FIGURE 5.5 *Image*

The full add power is achieved 16mm below the fitting cross. The corridor is 13.5mm in length. In addition to clear CR 39 plastic, it is available in a wide range of tints, including Transitions Gray, Brown, Transitions XTRActive Lenses, Nu Polar, Polarized Gray, and Polarized Brown. Additions are likely, and the local laboratory can be queried for updates.

Outlook (Vision-Ease Lens, Inc.)

The Outlook is one of the newer progressive addition designs with optics similar to those of the Image lens. The manufacturer identifies it as an aspheric, multi-design lens combining the best of hard and soft designs. A possible minimum fitting height of 18mm is compatible to the smaller fashion frames. It is man- ufactured in a polycarbonate called Tegra (Tegra is the trade name for Vision-Ease's polycarbonate lenses) and, in this design, is thin, light, and strong. The lens is also available in CR 39 plastic with a scratch-resistant coating (SR-CR 39) and in Transitions Gray. It is highly possible additional colors will be added. The local laboratory can be queried for updates.

VariVue (Vision-Ease Lens)

The VariVue is a soft PAL manufactured in crown glass, CR 39 plastic, high-index 1.56 plastic, identified as Thindex VariVue, and polycarbonate. It is described as a soft aspheric design. From the fitting cross to the lens edge, the minimum recommended measurement is 22mm. The glass design is also available in Photogray Extra and Photobrown Extra, which the manufacturer recommends as general-purpose lenses. The VariVue has the characteristics of other soft designs described earlier in this chapter and controls the "swimming" effect by limiting the size of the useable near area.

Gradal Top Progressives (Carl Zeiss Optical, Inc.)

The Gradal Top is described as an aspheric design, probably best interpreted as a multi-design PAL. This recently released lens will soon be available in a wide variety of materials. In addi- tion to conventional clear glass and a photochromic gray, the lens is manufactured in polycarbonate, index 1.59, and there- fore has all the benefits of being thin, light-weight, and almost unbreakable and absorbing 100% of harmful ultraviolet radiation. There is a prescription limitation from −6.00D to +4.50D, but this will be expanded in the near future.

The plastic Gradal Top, 1.67 index, is advertised as the slimmest progressive on the market, but there is limitation in prescription availability. It is also planned that the lens be manufactured with index 1.6 plastic, so the local laboratory needs to be contacted for updates.

Gradal RD (Carl Zeiss Optical, Inc.)

This CR 39 plastic lens is advertised as ideal for computer use. It has a wide progressive channel and a relatively wide reading area. However, to achieve this, there is considerable distortion surrounding these areas, so it is not recommended for general use. The manufacturer specifically cautions against wearing the lens while driving. The minimum fitting height should be 23mm to permit full use of the reading zone.

Percepta (Sola Optical USA)

The Percepta is advertised as having distorted areas in the lens that vary according to the base curve and power. The design, therefore, varies according to the prescription. From the fitting cross to the bottom of the lens, the measurement needs to be at least 22mm, but in the lower adds it can be 21mm. It is available in a number of materials; plastic CR 39, Transitions Gray, Transitions Brown, Transitions XTRActive, polycarbonate, and a high-index plastic called Finalite 1.6 (which makes for an extremely thin lens). There is also a high-index glass, 1.6. There is a Percepta in Polaroid (plastic). The decision to prescribe these lenses depends on the preference of the practitioner. Customizing a lens according to prescription may hold a certain appeal.

VIP (Sola Optical USA)

The VIP lens has a relatively wide near useable area, so distortion is intense in the lower periphery of the lens. It basically is a hard design. The vertical dimension of the frame must allow for a minimum of 22mm from the fitting cross (usually coinciding with the center of the pupil) to the bottom of the lens. It is available in CR 39 plastic, a high-index plastic called VIP Gold, polycarbonate, and in a number of Transitions tints. Glass photochromic designs also are manufactured.

XL (Sola Optical USA)

This PAL is a softer design than the VIP. It has a wide, clear intermediate area but a narrower near field. It is recommended for lower add prescriptions and can be fit with 21mm minimum from the fitting cross to the bottom of the lens. It is available in CR 39 plastic, a high-index plastic called XL Gold, polycarbonate, glass photochromic, and some shades of Transitions.

Access (Sola Optical USA)

The Access is unlike other PALs in that it has no distance prescription. It is designed for computer use and features progressive adds through an intermediate corridor until the full add is reached. When ordering, no height is given, only the near P.D. A frame must be selected that allows the vertical dimension of the finished lens to be at least 30mm. It may be advisable to select an adjustable pad frame. This allows for any necessary adjustments so that it meets perfectly the patient's needs while using a computer. It is manufactured in CR 39 and polycarbonate and can be tinted if glare from the screen is annoying to the patient.

Progressive Addition Lenses with Personalized Trade Names

It has been noted that a number of local eyecare centers are advertising PALs under their own specific trade name. It is easy to identify the lens as a soft design or a hard design by listening to the radio or television announcer. If the explanation says the lens offers a wide near area free of distortion, it is a hard design. The announcer may also say it is designed for use while working on computers. It is a soft design when advertised as minimum distortion and can be worn while walking. (Those having multi-design optics are difficult to identify from the announcer's text.)

Obviously, the advertiser is buying the lens from a major manufacturer/distributor and applying a trade-name for sales purposes. (Advertising for polycarbonate lenses with exclusive trade names has been done for a number of years.) Fitting procedures that are compatible to the optics of the lens (explained earlier in this chapter) are in order, but it must be remembered that regardless of design, some patients cannot adjust to the distorted areas.

IMPORTANT CONSIDERATIONS
REGARDING ALL PROGRESSIVE ADDITION LENSES

1. Extra foveal vision is disturbed by lateral aberration zones, so eye movements are restricted. There can be disturbances in binocular vision. To some degree this is controlled by an accurate monocular P.D. and by measuring each eye vertically from the center of the pupil to lower lens edge in normal illumination. This measurement must be 22mm or higher, unless prescribing a design in which this can be altered. For example, PALs meant for narrowed frames (as described previously in this chapter) can be a minimum of 18mm for this measurement. When the finished prescription is received from the laboratory, the crosslines marked on every PAL are meant to coincide with the center of the pupil (except for the Access).

    Note: Manufacturers tend to recommend the use of a "trade-name" corneal reflection pupillometer for taking a monocular P.D. However, all models basically give the same reading.

2. Since the dividing lines found in conventional multifocals are absent, the lenses provide superior cosmetic benefits as well as optical advantages to the presbyope who wants clear vision in all eye/head positions. However, optical distortions and reduced near field limit their use. Measurements for progressive corridors and near areas can vary according to design/prescription. In all cases, manufacturers agree there are some variations on measurements given in catalogues. Clinically, it has been noted that the same design having different prescriptions can have some difference in the clear-zone areas. Another problem is that all manufacturers may not use the same reference points, so stated sizes are not as meaningful as they could be.

3. Lens measurements must be taken on the frame the patient will wear. A properly fitting bridge is critical in controlling slippage down the nose which can effect the clear-zone areas. It is best not to use frames with an obvious nasal cut (seen on most aviator designs). The best mountings for PALs are conservative in shape without being too wide horizontally.

4.   A large pantoscopic angle allows the patient to better "ignore" blur areas. Lower edges of the lenses/frame should be angled close to the cheeks. A secure adjustment is very important, so straight-back temples styles should not be dispensed. Skull and comfort cable designs help hold the eyewear in place.

5.   If a patient is already wearing PALs whose optics are in question, the lenses can be sent to the laboratory for identification. Manufacturers mark lenses with "signs" that can be interpreted by experts.

6.   Prism cannot be obtained by decentration and must be ground into PALs by the local laboratory.

7.   While PALs are available in a wide range of sphere, cylinder, and add corrections, there are some limits. If in doubt regarding a specific design, consult the local laboratory.

8.   Most manufacturers suggest an additional +0.25D add for near over that determined for a bifocal correction.

CONCLUSION

The decision as to which specific PAL to prescribe depends on the practitioner's professional judgment and the needs of the patient. Essentially, lenses having the same described optics are the same from every manufacturer/distributor. Every soft lens, for example, has its prescription "fed" into a computer and exhibits similar distorted areas for each trade name.

The "secret" to successful fitting is to fit the lenses so the patient reaches the same distorted areas in the right and left lens as he or she looks down. Taking the measurements in the manner described earlier in this chapter is *critical*. PALs will be replaced (at no charge) by almost every distributor with a conventional bifocal/trifocal if the patient cannot adjust to the distorted areas.

While this chapter outlines the basics of the more widely advertised PALs, there are dozens of manufacturers/distributors in the United States. In 1986 "invisible" multifocals captured only about 7% to 8% of the total multifocal market. There was a relatively equal division between blended/Seamless bifocals and PALs (statistic from the U.S. Optical Manufacturers' National Consumer Eyewear Survey). In late 1999 to early 2000, the figure is closer to 20% for PALs alone.

While blended (Seamless) bifocals appear to have found a steady market, the use of PALs has a direct correlation between educational programs and sales figures. Seminars sponsored by manufacturers to acquaint eyecare professionals with specific designs are given frequently. They are a "must" for manufacturers needing a share of the PAL market.

For patients who will not wear multifocals "with lines," "invisible" designs are needed. While PALs are promoted for allowing clear vision at all distances, in reality, most patients seek the lenses for cosmetic reasons; they associate conventional multifocals with maturity.

Patients requesting "invisible" multifocals are usually more satisfied when the lenses are prescribed in conjunction with a utilitarian correction. For instance, a flat-top 28mm bifocal is preferred for an 8-hour-a-day job, but eyewear having more cosmetic value is wanted for dress occasions. Others may find the peripheral distortion unacceptable for driving a car yet welcome a PAL design while shopping, because almost every object can be seen clearly through some portion of the lens. The gradual power change also eliminates double images, which are often annoying to wearers of conventional bifocals/trifocals.

Manufacturers sometimes hesitate to use the terms *hard structure* and *soft structure* to describe the optics of their designs. (A hard-structure lens has peripheral distortion that is highly concentrated. The soft-structure design spreads out peripheral distortion; the hope is that it will be less annoying to the wearer. The newer term, *multi-design,* can indicate a compromise between a hard and soft design.) Studying the material supplied with every PAL design is an absolute *must.* It gives an excellent clue as to prescribing possibilities.

It is *most important* to order PALs from a laboratory that has the expertise to process them correctly. This is a critical consideration in maintaining the optics described by the manufacturer and in accordance to the specifications of the practitioner.

Chapter 6

PRESCRIBING DOUBLE-SEGMENT AND QUADRIFOCAL LENSES

INTRODUCTION

Double-segment lenses are designed for presbyopic patients whose vocational and/or avocational needs involve seeing objects clearly both above eye level and at the customary reading distance. The lenses feature a lower segment that has an add power almost always determined at the normal reading position and an upper segment usually focused at about arm's length. Patients most likely to benefit from double-segment lenses include eyecare professionals, pharmacists, librarians, in-store salespersons, postal clerks, and dentists, among others. A careful case history is the best guide to prescribing this lens design.

DOUBLE-SEGMENT GLASS LENSES

It is highly recommended that double-segment lenses be prescribed in a plastic design. At one time, it was difficult to find suitable plastic designs for every occupational need, but now this is highly unlikely. The hard-resin CR 39 designs have expanded drastically, and a variety are made available from many optical manufacturers. However, since glass double-segment lenses are manufactured and often prescribed, availability is discussed in this chapter.

Double-segment lenses fashioned of glass are available in both fused and one-piece construction. Almost every style has an upper add power that is a fixed percentage of the near, usually 75%. For example, if the near add is +2.50D the upper intermediate add is +1.87D or $^3/_4$ of the near power. Some, however, have an add power that is the same for both segments, so it is important to query the local laboratory/manufacturer for specifics. The standard separation between the two segments is usually a fixed distance of 13mm or 14mm.

Double-segment glass lenses are manufactured in clear and in a wide variety of shades of pink, gray, and green. They are also available in Photogray Extra and Photobrown Extra. The specifics are ascertained by querying the manufacturer/local laboratory. However, with the wide availability of color lens coatings that have suitable absorption curves, ordering any desired color is not a problem.

Lenses that change color according to environmental needs (photochromics) are available in a number of double-segment glass designs. Almost all are Photogray Extra and Photobrown Extra, and updates on availability are offered by local optical laboratories. These lenses tend to be popular because people who work outdoors-indoors often find the color change capability very convenient.

The availability of standard double-segment designs has been greatly expanded in recent years. In addition, Vision-Ease Lens, the largest manufacturer of glass lenses in the United States, will custom make dual designs in fused segments to almost any prescription with almost any desired separation. The local laboratory should be queried for updated information about a specific need.

DESIGNS OF DOUBLE-SEGMENT LENSES

Flat-top Double D-25mm

At one time, this design, which features a conventional FT25mm D-style lower segment and an upper segment that is an inverted standard D-style 25mm, was one of the most widely prescribed double-segment lenses (Figure 6.1). The separation between the segments is almost always 13mm, but some manufacturers use 12mm and 14mm (check with the local laboratory for specifics). Laboratories can supply this lens in the same amount of time as any conventional multifocal when 13mm is the separation between the two segments.

Flat-top double D-25mm lenses are manufactured in a wide range of pink, gray, and green shades. (Color coatings can be applied to a clear lens for other choices.) For patients needing a photochromic lens, Photogray Extra and Photobrown Extra are available. Today, however, most eyecare professionals prefer recommending larger-segment designs such as the double D-28.

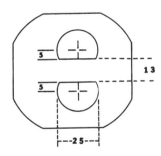

FIGURE 6.1 *Flat-top double D-25mm*

Flat-top Double D-28mm

Two FT28mm D-style segments are placed in the same position as in the double D-25mm (Figure 6.2). This lens is for patients needing relatively large near and upper intermediate areas, not unusual for occupations requiring double segments. This design now surpasses the popularity of the double D-25mm style. The standard separation is 13mm or 14mm, depending on the manufacturer. It is available in shades of pink, gray, and green (query the local laboratory for specifics), and color coatings on a clear lens expand the possibilities. Photogray Extra and Photobrown Extra remain popular choices for the outdoor-indoor worker.

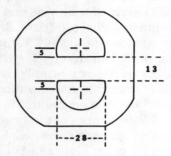

FIGURE 6.2   *Flat-top double D-28mm*

Flat-top Double D-35 Segments

This unusually wide-segment flat-top double D-35mm design is an excellent recommendation for presbyopes needing critical vision for large areas at near and overhead seeing. The standard separation between the 35mm segments is 15mm (Figure 6.3). The upper add power is not necessarily a certain percentage of the near because these are custom lenses (from Vision-Ease Lens). Specific working distances need to be determined and adds ordered that fill the patient's needs. It is available in many shades of pink, gray, and green as well as color coatings on a clear lens. Photogray Extra and Photobrown Extra are the photochromic designs. Since these lenses are custom designed, it is best to query the local laboratory as to delivery time.

Executive Double Segment

This one-piece design, introduced by American Optical, is not likely to be available much longer. It features segments separated by straight lines extending from the nasal to the temporal extremities of the lens; the segments are 14mm apart (Figure 6.4). The power of the upper portion is standard 75% of the near add. As with all lenses of this construction, the dividing lines have a pronounced "shelf," and when high adds are involved in the glass design, the outer limits tend to chip unless great care is exercised in handling. It was manufactured in Photogray

Extra and Photobrown Extra but was not standard in other colors.

Patients still wearing this lens should be prescribed another double-segment design. Probably the best is the double D-35 (DD-35). The standard separation is 15mm, but 16mm or 17mm is available on special order in glass from Vision-Ease Lens.

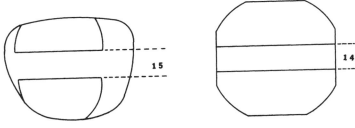

FIGURE 6.3 *Flat-top D-35mm*   FIGURE 6.4 *Executive double*

Double 22mm Round Top

Although this lens is still available, it is rarely recommended. The upper and lower segments of the fused design are 22mm round with a standard separation of 14mm. The lower segment is conventional in appearance; the other is inverted in the upper portion of the lens. Since the widest area of each segment is 11mm from the dividing line, it is obvious a great many head/neck movements are necessary to utilize the widest portion of the near and intermediate areas. Optical performance is more advantageous in previously discussed designs and should be seriously considered before this lens is prescribed.

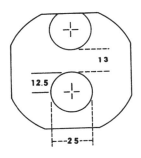

FIGURE 6.5 *Double 25mm round*

Double-round 25mm Segment

The double-round 25mm lens features two segments: a conventional 25mm round for the lower add and an inverted 25mm round for the upper segment. The standard separation is 13mm. (Appearance is similar to double-round 22mm but with larger segments.) (Figure 6.5) While it appears that this lens is not advantageous over the flat-top DD-25mm, it is still prescribed and even available with a 12mm, 14mm, 15mm, and a 16mm separation (check with the local laboratory for special orders). The same problems with head tilt, etc., that exist with the double-round 22mm segment are present with this design.

Double-round 28mm Segments

The lens features two 28mm round segments, a conventional 28mm round for the lower add and an inverted 28mm segment for the upper. Like the double-round 25mm, it has a standard 13mm separation but is available with a 14mm, 15mm, and 16mm separation. The flat-top DD-28mm lenses are a more optically sound choice for patients needing upper and lower adds.

Double-round 35 Segments

Two round 35mm segments are separated by 15mm standard. A smaller separation is not manufactured, but 16mm, 17mm, and even 18mm separations are available from Vision-Ease Lens on custom orders. It is far preferable to recommend a double-D (flat-top) 35mm design for patients needing large segments.

A possible explanation for the continuing use of double-round segments is their cosmetic value. The segments are far less prominent than the flat-top D designs. This appears to be a motivating factor primarily outside the United States because these lenses continue to be prescribed in other countries. Eyecare professionals in the United States almost overwhelmingly prescribe the double-D flat-top styles.

Note: While other double segment designs may be listed in catalogues, it is highly unlikely they are available or even necessary. Designs such as double A-style, double ribbon segments, serve no useful purpose and are probably listed only to enhance the "availability list" of a manufacturer.

PLASTIC CR 39 DOUBLE-SEGMENT LENSES

It is highly recommended that plastic CR 39 lenses be recommended whenever feasible. While the index of 1.49 makes them thicker than glass (distance index 1.523), they are much safer, and since they are occupational lenses, the added thickness is not likely to be a cosmetic factor.

CR 39 double segments are currently available in many designs that are comparable with glass. However, unlike the glass designs, manufacturers will not make special orders (which are rarely necessary anyway) that vary from stated specifications.

Double Flat-top D-25mm, CR 39

Like its glass counterpart, this design is being replaced by the larger segments more suitable for occupational use. The separation between the two segments is a standard 13mm with the upper add 75% of the near. Its appearance is the same as the glass flat-top D-25mm described previously in this chapter.

Double Flat-top D-28mm, CR 39

This is the usually recommended double-segment lens. The two standard D-style segments are separated by 14mm. The upper add is 75% of the near (illustration of glass design applies here).

Double Flat-top 35mm (Dual 35) CR 39

The double flat-top 35mm (dual 35) CR 39 lens is a relatively new segment design. The lower segment is a flat-top 35mm, the upper an inverted flat-top 35mm. The standard separation is 15mm. It is an excellent occupational double-segment design, supplying a wide near and wide upper intermediate field. It should be seriously considered for most occupational uses.

Double Executive Segments

Like the glass counterpart, this lens is not likely to be available. The segments extend across the entire lens. There is a narrow distance corridor that is 14mm high. The power of the upper segment is 75% of the near. The thick shelves of the CR

39 material make this an unsightly lens. A patient needing large segments should be able to use the dual 35mm (double flat-top DD) efficiently.

Note: As of this writing, double-segment lenses in polycarbonate plastic are not manufactured. This may change in the near future.

FITTING PROCEDURE

It is important that double-segment lenses be positioned correctly so the patient can utilize them properly. The fitting procedure outlined here is offered as a guide.

Since positioning the two segments is critical, minute changes in frame adjustment often determine patient satisfaction. It is almost always best to dispense a frame having an adjustable-pad bridge construction. (Eye practitioners sometimes visit an on-site location to help the patient determine actual optical needs.)

1.   Using the *exact frame* that has been selected, measure the vertical dimension (be sure to add for the lens bevel if a rimmed frame is involved).

2.   Placing the frame on the patient's face, determine the height of the lower segment (usually the dividing line is positioned at the lower lid for a flat-top segment; slightly higher for a round-top).

3.   Add the distance separating the two segments—usually 13 or 14mm—to the height of the lower segment.

4.   The remaining lens area will be the height of the upper segment. To create a comfortable, usable area of vision, this measurement needs to be a minimum of 9mm. If it is not, a frame having more vertical should be dispensed. In some instances, it may be feasible to position the lower segment slightly lower than usual to allow more area in the upper segment.

QUADRIFOCALS

It is possible to prescribe a lens that has an inverted bifocal segment over a trifocal design, identified as a quadrifocal (Figure 6.6). Such a lens can bring added visual efficiency to the older

ity need to be checked with the local laboratory because there is relatively little demand for A-style segments.

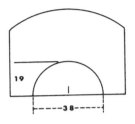

FIGURE 7.9   *Ultex A style*

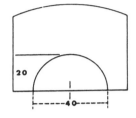

FIGURE 7.10   *Wide seg-40*

Wide Seg-40 Round (40mm × 20mm)

The positioning of the optical center of this segment, 20mm below the dividing line, is comparable with that of the glass King-Size Ultex (Figure 7.10). The high amount of image jump limits its use; large straight-top segments that have optical centers close to or at the dividing line are preferable occupational bifocals.

Curved Top with Sharp Corners

The glass counterpart is the original Tillyer Sovereign. Several plastic bifocals similar in appearance have been distributed in the United States, but they are rarely seen. Vision-Ease Lens lists C25 and C28 as available in CR 39 (Figure 7.11) but the best choice for these sizes are the D style 25mm and 28mm.

CR 39 TRIFOCAL DESIGNS

There are available CR 39 trifocal designs that meet the needs of presbyopes requiring specific-size intermediate segments. Like bifocals, they are manufactured in one-piece minus-cylinder form. The standard near adds range in power from +1.50D to +3.00D, depending on the design (the local laboratory can be queried for specifics), with a standard intermediate power that is 50% of the near addition. Vision-Ease also makes several designs with intermediate segment powers 40%, 60%, and 70% of the near add, but availability for a specific prescription should be checked.

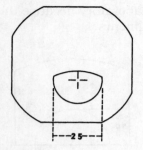

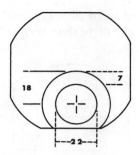

FIGURE 7.11   *Curved-top (C)*

FIGURE 7.12   *Round-top trifocal (discontinued)*

Round-top Trifocal (Discontinued)

The round-top trifocal featured a 22mm round near segment surrounded by an intermediate circular band of 7mm (Figure 7.12). It was the first trifocal manufactured in CR 39 plastic. Since the straight-top designs offer more efficiency and optical value, this lens has been discontinued. Patients wearing this lens need to be given a straight-top trifocal.

Straight-top (Flat-top) 7mm × 25mm Trifocal

This is the most widely prescribed trifocal in both glass and plastic. Straight dividing lines separate the intermediate segment from the distance area and the intermediate from the near. The intermediate is a band 7mm high; the near segment is a straight-top D-style bifocal (rounded lower extremities). Adequate viewing areas are provided for most patients, and a relatively pleasing cosmetic appearance is maintained (Figure 7.13). The CR 39 design is made with the standard 50% intermediate segment power. The glass counterpart can be ordered with an intermediate power 40%, 60%, or 70% of the near add.

Note: The original ST6-22, CR 39 trifocal has been phased out because of the limited size segment areas.

Straight-top 7mm × 28mm

Comparable in appearance to the ST7-25 trifocal, this lens is prescribed with increased frequency (Figure 7.14). Many patients enjoy the wider near and intermediate areas; 28mm allows for a comfortable near field. It is manufactured in the standard 50% intermediate power.

Note: The ST7-25 and ST7-28 plastic trifocals are appropriate designs when a bicentric correction is indicated. The slab-off line is customarily placed to coincide with the division between the intermediate and near segments (Figure 7.15). Reverse slab-off may not be available.

Straight-top 7mm × 35mm

Designed for the patient needing an exceptionally wide near area, the 35mm near segment results in a popular occupational trifocal (Figure 7.16). As with all large-segment lenses, the dividing lines are relatively pronounced but not as obvious as those in the straight-across trifocal design. This lens can be used for slab-off corrections.

Note: Vision-Ease Lens also makes this design with an 8mm high intermediate segment listed as 8 TRI 35 (comparable to straight-top 8-35).

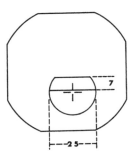

FIGURE 7.13 *Straight-top 7-25*

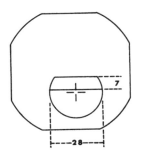

FIGURE 7.14 *Straight-top 7-28*

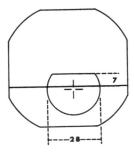

FIGURE 7.15 *Slab-off straight-top 7-28*

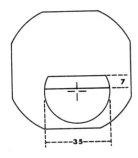

FIGURE 7.16 *Straight-top 7-35*

DATALITE TRIFOCAL FOR VDT USERS

In 1986 Vision-Ease Lens released the Datalite trifocal for wear at video display terminals (VDTs). The lens is available in CR 39 hard resin only. The near add is a ST35mm segment; the intermediate segment measures 14mm high, giving an excellent vision area at the distance most VDTs are placed (Figure 7.17). The power, 66% of the lower add, was determined by research to give the best intermediate acuity. The lens exhibits UV-absorbing characteristics. Color compatible with the factory in-mold scratch-resistant coating can be ordered if the patient needs additional protection from glare.

Straight-across (Full-segment) Trifocals

This lens looks like an Executive glass trifocal. Both the near and intermediate segments extend to the extremities of the lens blank with the intermediate band measuring 7mm high (Figure 7.18). Therefore, the distance correction is limited to the upper portion of the lens. It is strictly a vocational design for patients needing unusually large and/or wide intermediate and near segments. Cosmesis is poor because of the obvious "shelves" of the dividing lines.

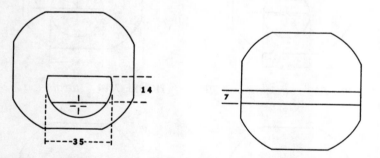

FIGURE 7.17   *Datalite trifocal—VDT*   **FIGURE 7.18**   *Straight-across trifocal*

Sola E/D Trifocal (Sola Worldwide)

As the initials E/D imply, the Sola E/D trifocal featured an Executive-style intermediate segment that extends from the temporal to the nasal extremities of the lens surrounding a 25mm straight-top D-style reading segment (Figure 7.19). It is manufactured in CR 39 plastic only. Introduced and manufactured in Europe, it never gained acceptance in the United States.

Univis Ultra CV (Continuous Vision; Discontinued)

This Ultra CV trifocal had a distinctive design best visualized by looking at Figure 7.20. The near segment is a 24mm D-style positioned inside an intermediate area measuring 28mm at the widest point.

Univis has discontinued all lens production, and no other manufacturer makes the design. Patients wearing this lens need to be prescribed another general-purpose trifocal. The ST7-25mm or ST7-28mm should prove satisfactory.

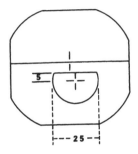

FIGURE 7.19 *Sola E/D (Executive/D-style segments)*

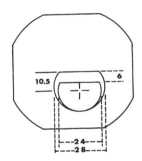

FIGURE 7.20 *Univis Ultra CV—CR 39 (discontinued)*

DOUBLE-SEGMENT OCCUPATIONAL CR 39 LENSES

Double-segment lenses, characterized by upper and lower adds separated by the distance prescription and designed to give the patient an add power for overhead seeing, are available in CR 39 plastic. These are discussed in Chapter 6 "Prescribing Double-Segment and Quadrifocal Lenses." People whose occupations require this kind of clarity, including pharmacists, dentists, and showroom salespeople, often prefer the lightness of plastic to the glass designs. The distance area is limited to the separation between the two segments (the standard is 13mm or 14mm, depending on the CR 39 design), so these lenses are prescribed in addition to conventional eyewear. The procedure for positioning double segments is explained in Chapter 6, "Prescribing Double-Segment and Quadrifocal Lenses."

PROGRESSIVE ADDITION LENSES

There are a number of progressive addition lenses available in CR 39 plastic. They are explained in Chapter 5 "Prescribing 'Invisible' Multifocals." However, a special design called Varilux Overview is discussed here because its use is the same as a double-segment lens.

Varilux Overview

The lower portion of the Varilux Overview is a progressive addition design. The upper area carries a 41mm bifocal shaped like a half moon (Figure 7.21). The upper add power is always 0.50D less than the full add. This lens has limited use. While the upper add is without distortion, there is distortion in the periphery of the rest of the lens. Professional judgment and a careful case history are important before prescribing. To give an adequate viewing upper area, a deep frame pattern that allows a 10mm to 12mm segment height is necessary. The upper segment division probably is best placed at the upper edge of the pupil in normal illumination.

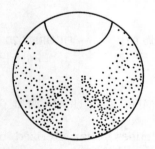

FIGURE 7.21   *Varilux Overview*

POLYCARBONATE PLASTIC LENSES

It is highly recommended that polycarbonate plastic lenses be prescribed whenever possible. They are vastly superior to both glass and CR 39 plastic. In fact, polycarbonate plastic lenses with the high index of 1.586 are the fastest-growing lens market for a number of excellent reasons (discussed in this chapter). In the near future, it is expected that they will be the overwhelming choice of both eyecare providers and patients.

Few companies actually manufacture polycarbonates, but every major lens distributor includes polycarbonate lenses in their inventory and distributes them under its own trade name. Gentex, the largest manufacturer, distributes the lenses under the name Profile. Other recognizable trade names include the following:

Omega	Life Style
Essilor	Thin and Light
Vision-Ease Lens	Tegra

Usually each local laboratory stocks one brand of polycarbonates and supplies it for all prescriptions. Basically, the optical properties of each are the same, so it may be a waste of time (and not necessary) to specify a company's name.

Polycarbonate lenses are advertised extensively on radio and television by local eyecare practitioners and optical companies under their own trade names. There can be hundreds of these names in the United States, but the lenses are recognized as polycarbonates by the announcer's description, such as, virtually unbreakable so should be prescribed for children (about 50% of children needing eyewear in the United States wear these lenses—it should be closer to 100%), cosmetically attractive, thinner than conventional lenses, beautifully mounted into modern frame designs, and so forth. Eyecare professionals in shopping malls throughout the United States also use advertising posters, etc., depicting beautiful people wearing the attractive polycarbonate lenses (a great service to the public), but identified by their trademark name rather than "polycarbonate."

Advantages of Polycarbonate Lenses

1. **Virtually unbreakable.** The lens is like a bullet-proof shield for the eyes. This is an invaluable asset for all children, persons involved in active sports, monocular and partially sighted patients in whose care every precaution must be taken to preserve the remaining vision. (Actually, everyone can benefit from polycarbonate lenses because one never knows when an accident involving the eyes or vision may occur.)

2. **Absorption of all harmful ultraviolet radiations.** Since the ozone layer that protects the earth from UV rays is being depleted, eyes need this protection to

prevent ocular pathological conditions that can occur from exposure to the sun, such as snow blindness and early cataracts. These lenses block both harmful UVA and UVB rays by 99% to 99.9% (discussed in Chapter 9 "Prescribing Absorptive Lenses").

3. **Lightness.** Polycarbonate lenses are so light they can feel almost weightless on the face. In all cases, they are lighter than CR 39 by about 10% and much, much lighter than glass (by 55% to 60%).

4. **High scratch and abrasion resistance.** Hardness coatings are applied on both surfaces by the manufacturers. It is recommended that antireflection coatings also be ordered. Uncoated, the lenses have 89% light transmission; antireflection coatings bring light transmission to 99.5%. This makes for reduction of ghost images and flaring of lights, a great advantage when operating a motor vehicle, especially at night. There is also a great cosmetic advantage; when reflections are drastically reduced, the eyes and eye area are more visible to the onlooker.

5. **Tints** have become more stable, especially in the darker shades, almost eliminating the major problems of the past. Suntints such as gray no. 2 and gray no. 3, the most widely recommended shades, tend to stay true for a very long period of time.

6. **These are beautiful lenses.** The high index allows for a thinner lens with flatter curves. The resultant eyewear, particularly in the higher powers, is a joy for the wearer.

Polycarbonate lenses do have a few disadvantages. Sometimes in high powers, because of the higher index, there is some noticeable color aberration in the periphery. However, with the fashion trend toward smaller eyeframes, this is rarely a problem. They are not manufactured in some very high powers. There is also a limitation in multifocal designs, but most prescriptions are available in a flat-top 25mm bifocal and a straight-top (flat-top) 25mm bifocal. Trifocals are manufactured in a straight-top 7.28 and ST 8-35 with an intermediate power 50% of the near.

Progressive addition polycarbonate lens designs are also now available. These are discussed in Chapter 5 "Prescribing 'Invisible' Multifocals." Local laboratories should be contacted frequently for updated information.

At one time, some optical laboratories did not process poly-carbonates (more skill required, special equipment, etc.) but this is rarely the case today. As polycarbonates move toward capturing a larger share of the lens market, every local labora-tory will be prepared for the expansion. Polycarbonates are the lenses of the future.

OTHER HIGH INDEX PLASTIC LENSES

A number of optical catalogues list high-index plastic lenses identified as *high-index CR 39.* These lenses, which have an index over 1.586 (usually 1.6 or 1.7), are not necessarily supe-rior to polycarbonates. While in theory the slightly high index means a "thinner" lens, practically speaking, this difference is rarely discernable to the eye. A possible disadvantage may be that the slightly higher index results in more chromatic aberra-tion, but in actuality the difference is so slight it may not be dis-cernable to the patient.

High-index CR 39 lenses may not have the comparable impact resistance of polycarbonates nor the inherent ultraviolet protection. Depending on the manufacturer, they may not be as scratch resistant (although a scratch resistant coating can be applied). It probably is always best to prescribe polycarbonates whenever the needed prescription/lens design is available.

Chapter 8

OPHTHALMIC LENS COATINGS

INTRODUCTION

Undoubtedly, one of the most remarkable additions to the lens design field during the past decade is the development and increased use of coatings applied to surfaces of both glass and plastic lenses. They can enhance fashion tinting, are available in tones that absorb radiation harmful to the eye, and, when applied in antireflection form, make direct and reflected light less bothersome to the wearer.

While these coatings when applied correctly can greatly enhance the enjoyment of the eyewear (specifics noted later in this chapter), with failure to use proper lens blanks (e.g., base curves for a certain prescription) or proven coating techniques, the coatings may crack, peel, and/or make the lens difficult to clean. Probably the only way to know for sure the quality of the coating/process is communication with the laboratory. The best-designed lens for a given prescription to which the coating will be placed is critical. Equipment is also important. Outdated or poorly designed equipment will not produce quality coatings.

The laboratory must clean the lenses meticulously before applying the coatings to insure proper adhesion. Some lenses received from the factory have the scratch-resistant coating on the front side only. In that case, it is important to also order a quality hard coating on the back surface. Improved patient satisfaction makes the extra cost well worth the advantages.

COATINGS FOR GLASS LENSES

While the increased use of plastic lenses is slowly making obsolete glass lenses (in the United States) except for certain prescriptions not available in plastic, this chapter will first discuss coatings for glass lenses because these were the original and are still recommended in many parts of the United States and the world.

There are available several types of coatings that when applied to glass lenses offer specific advantages to the patient. These coatings are not to be confused with the coatings for CR 39 plastic, polycarbonate lenses, and some high-index plastic lenses that result in a hard, abrasion-resistant surface (discussed later). The glass coating most commonly prescribed is an antireflection layer applied to both surfaces of the lens. The process makes it possible to eliminate approximately two-thirds of the reflections normally noted on crown lenses and about three-fourths of those ordinarily seen on high-index glass.

Since a lens is visible because of reflected light from its surfaces, an antireflection coating offers several cosmetic advantages. When clear lenses are coated properly, they can appear almost invisible. The eyes and eye area are seen in better perspective, thus allowing for more expressive interest in the face.

Coatings for glass lenses are also available in a wide variety of colors. These tints are applied either to the front or the back surface or to both surfaces, depending on the professional judgment of the manufacturer. An antireflection coating that reduces reflections is usually then applied over the color coating.

A coating of a protective nature, sometimes referred to as a *permanent layer,* is also available. It is placed over color and antireflection coatings to help keep them intact.

ANTIREFLECTION COATINGS ON GLASS LENSES

When a beam of light strikes a clear ophthalmic glass lens, light transmission is about 92%. The remaining 8% is lost through reflections from the front and back surfaces of the lens. Although this loss of light can result in a slight decrease in visual acuity, the problem usually encountered by the patient is awareness of annoying reflections. Modern antireflection coatings can increase light transmission to as much as 98% in some lenses.

An antireflection coating is composed of $1/4$ of a wavelength of magnesium fluoride. While it is a physical impossibility to coat a lens to be completely free of a tinge of color, the index of magnesium fluoride (about 1.36) allows a crown lens to appear almost colorless when applied by a skilled technician. However, this coating may still show a slight purplish cast because a single layer of magnesium fluoride does not allow for the red and blue light to be completely cancelled. A better choice is ordering multilayer coatings. They cancel reflected light over a wide band of colors, so the coated lens surface tends to be free of the characteristic purplish cast.

Some practitioners recommend antireflection coatings on all prescribed glass lenses. However, the following patients may benefit more than others when this coating is used:

1. **Patients concerned about the annoyance of reflected light when driving at night.** In dim illumination, reflections of bright objects such as oncoming headlights are often manifested as double images. In many cases, the driver's judgment as to distance and other vision-related factors is adversely affected. Antireflection coatings provide a more comfortable environment, making it safer to drive at night.

2. **Patients wearing a correction of –2.00D or greater.** The presence of myopic rings is a major cosmetic disadvantage with glass minus lenses. These internal reflections are considerably reduced with the use of an antireflection coating. (It is important to remember, however, that polycarbonate plastic lenses are a far better cosmetic choice for minus corrections.)

3. **Patients wearing high-power plus lenses.** When high plus glass lenses are worn, the ghost images reflected from the lens surfaces, although rather vague, are relatively large and can be very annoying. An antireflection coating reduces this source of irritation and improves the appearance of the eyewear. (A far better choice for high plus lenses are aspheric plastic designs that dramatically improve appearance and reduce the weight of the lenses.)

4. **Patients wearing high-power prism lenses.** If the prism power is high enough for a noticeable difference in edge thickness, the lenses are a cosmetic problem. Since reflections from the surfaces of a prism are also pronounced, coating the lenses helps their appearance. (Again, polycarbonates are a far better choice.)

5. **Any patient wearing glasses who is concerned about ghost images and/or light reflections.** There are sensitive patients who are bothered by lens reflections even when the correction is low in power. Often they are wearers of multifocals, particularly concerned about reflections at the segment dividing lines. While some glass manufacturers attempt to solve the problem by coating the dividing lines of fused segments, the best results are achieved when the entire lens is treated with an antireflection coating. (Again, one-piece plastic multifocals are a better choice.)

Note: Antireflection coatings are sometimes confused with pink tints. Somehow, there is a mistaken perception that they solve the same problem, probably because both are recommended for reduction of glare. An antireflection coating allows more light to enter the eye; a tinted lens reduces light transmission. If there is a desire to reduce both lens reflections and light transmission, a pink no. 2 tint with an antireflection coating can be recommended. Light transmission through such a lens is approximately 89%.

Antireflection coatings are available from hundreds of optical suppliers. While some companies may use ordinary single-layer or two-layer coatings, a unique multilayered coating that allows over 99% of light to go through a clear lens (compared to about 96% with two-layer coatings and 92% with uncoated clear glass lenses) is by far the better choice.

Manufacturers may use from three to nine layers, but efficiency is not necessarily related to the number of layers. The selection of materials for refractive index, thickness with which the layers are applied, and the adherence capability to the previous layer are all factors. Interestingly, depending on all factors, the difference in percentage of light transmission may be slight, but patients report improved vision and lowered eye fatigue when the best is supplied.

COLOR COATINGS FOR GLASS LENSES

Metal oxide coatings in almost any desired color can be applied to glass lenses. There are several advantages to ordering lenses tinted by this method. When a suntint prescription other than plano is involved, glass lenses manifest a color difference from center to edge. This difference is barely perceptible in prescriptions under plus or minus 2.00D. When the prescription is over plus or minus 4.00D, the difference is almost always obvious enough that a method of color control is necessary (see Chapter 9, "Prescribing Absorptive Lenses"). One of these methods involves coating the lenses the desired shade. Since the color is applied evenly over the lens surface, it is always uniform (unless otherwise ordered, a gradient effect, for example).

When tinted glass lenses are wanted to create a fashion effect, the best method in obtaining these tints is usually the coating procedure. Almost any hue can be ordered, whereas conventional tints obtained by adding an oxide to the ingredients of clear glass are extremely limited. Suppliers of color coatings make available sample kits and provide accurate absorption curves (one coating company advertises more than 100 varieties). This allows the practitioner to also know the transmission properties of ultraviolet (UV) and infrared (IR) radiation. (Transmission of the visible spectrum can often be determined easily with the naked eye by looking through the colored lens at a known color. If the color changes, then obviously the visible spectrum is affected.) It is important not to use colors that affect interpretation of red/green/amber traffic lights. Unfortunately, rock stars and other entertainers sometimes make certain deep colors (e.g., purple) popular. Patients must be warned not to wear such lenses while operating a motor vehicle.

Note: A possible disadvantage of a color-coated lens was the slight metallic look that some patients found objectionable. However, newer processes involved in the coating procedure of glass lenses have considerably reduced this problem.

Coatings can be ordered to create special effects. The coating most requested gives a mirrored finish to the front surface. This mirror coating can be applied over any color, but mirror coatings over yellow, gray, brown, or green tints are the most popular. Lenses that are coated so that the upper portion is a deeper color than the lower (single gradient density lenses) or the upper and lower parts of the lenses are the deep color (double gradient density lenses) often have mirror coatings for a fashion effect. Manufacturers claim these special coatings reduce abnormal overhead glare and excessive brightness from "shiny" surfaces such as water, sand, or snow, but "in truth" their popularity tends to come and go depending on the whims of celebrities who wear them.

It has become common practice to include antireflection layers on color-coated lenses. This is an excellent advantage because reducing lens reflections adds to the attractiveness of the eyewear.

PROTECTIVE LAYERS FOR ANTIREFLECTION AND COLOR COATINGS ON GLASS LENSES

At one time, the principal disadvantage of wearing glass lenses treated with antireflection and color coatings was the difficulty encountered in keeping them clean. The coatings attracted dust and dirt. If the lens was wiped when dry or cleaned with silicone papers, abrasive material could mar the coatings. (The recommendation is always to run water over the lenses to wash away debris before drying.)

A durable hard layer has been developed that when applied over an antireflection and/or color coating almost eliminates this problem and allows the lenses to be cleaned by any conventional method. However, it is still best to wash the lenses whenever possible because that insures a smear-free surface.

Some laboratories place this protective layer over all antireflection and color coatings; others supply it only when ordered. It is important to be specific; the advantages offered by the protective layer are such that it should always be included. In addition to easier cleaning, it also helps prevent "peeling off" of the other coatings.

COATINGS FOR PLASTIC LENSES

It is likely that within the next decade, plastic lenses (CR 39, polycarbonates, and other high-index lenses) will replace almost all glass lenses in the United States The original problems in providing a scratch-resistant surface have been almost eliminated. There is now wide availability of specific scratch-resistant coatings for all plastic lenses. While proper cleaning in itself (holding the lenses under running water before wiping clean) keeps the surfaces from being marred, practitioners often hesitated to prescribe the plastic designs, especially CR 39 hard resin, which could scratch relatively easily. Newer coatings take care of most of the problems of the past.

Two processes made available in the United States in the early 1970s at about the same time—Hi-Quartz by Hoya Lens (this scratch-resistant coating was first used in Japan) and Diamond-film by Berg Industries—made possible the advances we have today. Originally, the coating was placed only on the convex surface of the lens. In 1979, it became possible to order the coating on both surfaces, theoretically making CR 39 as easy to clean as a glass lens. However, both the original Hoya and Berg coatings could crack if subjected to high heat. Frame adjustments requiring heat often had to be made with the lenses out of the mountings, a most difficult task at best. In desert communities such as Palm Springs, California, patients reported that the lenses "crackled" and had to be replaced if worn out-of-doors on exceptionally hot days.

Today widely available factory-coated, abrasion-resistant CR 39 lenses are generally very satisfactory. The coating is placed by some manufacturers on the outside surface only and by others on both surfaces. A wide range of single-vision and multifocal prescriptions are suitable for the procedure.

Originally, these were identified as *in-mold* coatings, meaning that the lens can be easily tinted to any desired shade (surmounting a problem with the original coatings). The color was consistent, eliminating the blotchy color streaking sometimes seen with the original. Color did not build up at the segment dividing lines of multifocals. Factory-applied coatings to plastic lenses are now so sophisticated that they are usually guaranteed to stay intact for the lifetime of the lens (hard coatings applied by the local laboratory to CR 39 lenses may not be as satisfactory).

While scratch-resistant coatings on CR 39 lenses are not prescribed primarily as antireflection coatings, they result in an increase in antireflection properties as well as light transmission. Clear CR 39 uncoated lenses transmit about 93% of incident light. This increases to about 96% when a scratch-resistant coating is applied.

Originally there were problems in achieving certain hues in tinted lenses having scratch-resistant layers. A solution has been found, and all available colors for a single vision lens can be accurately reproduced. However, there are a few multifocal hard-resin designs that cannot be coated satisfactorily. It is best to query the local laboratory when in doubt. It is also necessary to keep in mind that since the hard coatings are protective, a tinted CR 39 lens cannot be bleached and retinted a different shade or another color (color change is a simple procedure on uncoated CR 39 lenses).

Scratch-resistant coatings have great value when used on CR 39 aphakic lenses. Fortunately, implant cataract lens surgery has rendered these high-plus lenses almost obsolete in the United States. However, the typical cataract patient of the past is elderly and tends to fall asleep while wearing spectacles, which then fall off the face. If the bulbous outside surface contacts rough surfaces, unprotected lenses can easily scratch.

Note: All polycarbonate plastic lenses have scratch-resistant coatings placed on both surfaces at the factory level. These are discussed in Chapter 7, "Plastic Ophthalmic Lenses."

SOME SPECIFIC TRADE-NAME COATINGS FOR PLASTIC LENSES (CR 39, POLYCARBONATES, HI-INDEX DESIGNS)

There are some specific coatings for plastic lenses that are widely advertised to the eyecare professional. One of these is Crizal coated plastic lenses by Essilor of America, Inc. Crizal coatings can be applied to CR 39 plastic, to polycarbonates (identified as Airwear Plastic), to Aspherics (As), and Transitions lenses. Most of these coatings are processed on the factory level but some single-vision prescriptions are supplied to local laboratories to insure faster delivery time.

Crizal coatings are two-sided, anti-scratch (front and back surfaces) with an antireflection layer. There is an additional hydrophobic coating for easier cleaning. This cushion coating is a necessity for the As (Aspheric lens) with a 1.0 center so that it can pass the U.S. Food and Drug Administration (FDA) ruling for impact resistance. It helps absorb and dissipate some of the impact energy that may interfere with the ability of the lens to pass this test.

Generally speaking, however, the hydrophobic coating is applied to all lenses for easier cleaning. Antireflection coatings are relatively soft and tend to scratch easily. Greasy make-up and other smudges can be a problem. To increase the hardness and make the lens surfaces easier to clean, hydrophobic coatings (a special layer of silicon) were developed. The silicon deposit causes water and grease to form small droplets that are easy to wipe away yet do not effect antireflection properties.

Essilor guarantees the integrity of all Crizal coated lenses for a "lifetime," which is identified as the length of time the patient wears the original prescription.

Another widely promoted lens coating system available is from Carl Zeiss Optical Inc. (Zeiss takes credit for inventing the modern antireflection [AR] coating in 1935, although it took decades before it was widely used on ophthalmic lenses.) Advertisements in professional journals identify coating machine, B-12/IV, which uses an exclusive quartz glass bell jar during the coating process. The result is satisfactory coatings, particularly on specialized lenses such as phototropic, photochromic, and laminated designs.

Zeiss also concentrates on some specifics. A foundation coating is advertised as the hardest coating available for polycarbonates and other high-index plastic lenses. It will not yellow, even with extended exposure to UV rays, as do some other coatings. The drawback is that the lens cannot be tinted over the coating.

A specialty coating from Zeiss is identified as Cool Blue. This is a "fashion blue" mirror coating on the front surface of the lens with an antireflection multilayer coating on the back surface. These lenses reduce incoming light by 85% and provide 100% protection against UV radiation. Available in almost any prescription, they may be desired by those interested in a "high fashion" sunlens look.

Zeiss particularly stresses that their coatings be used on Transitions lenses. These plastic photochromic lenses perform best with antireflection coatings, and Zeiss contends that theirs outperform many others on the market.

The importance of every step in successful antireflection coating procedures is stressed—quality of lens surface, proper washing of the lens, application of a hydrophobic coating for easy cleaning. Zeiss offers a great service by emphasizing these guidelines repeatedly in their literature to the eyecare professional.

EDGE COATINGS FOR MINUS LENSES

The local laboratory can apply color edge coatings on CR 39 high-minus or prism lenses to eliminate the opaqueness of the bevels. While color edge coatings are available for glass lenses, they are rarely used because glass bevels do not have an opaque look. The best effect is achieved when the coating is a light shade matching a light rimmed frame (the dark shades give a "tunnel" effect to the eyewear, e.g., black plastic frame, black edge coating).

Edge coatings are usually applied by hand with a small brush then hardened in an oven with a controlled temperature. The result depends on the skill and care of the technician, but experience shows that patients often are displeased even with the best effect. They do not necessarily improve the cosmetic appearance of the eyewear, so it is always best to show a sample to the patient before ordering.

Much better solutions for attractive high-minus/prism lenses are polycarbonate or higher-index plastic lenses tinted a soft hue. The palest pink tone is the most popular because it blends with all skin tones and is appropriate for both men and women.

CONCLUSION

A great number of lens coatings manufacturers (for both glass and plastic lenses) operate in the United States. Only a very few are mentioned here. Basically the best source of information is the local laboratory that either processes the lenses or sends them to the manufacturer's factory for processing. Quality on the local level varies greatly. It is critical that the eyecare practitioner have confidence in the coatings supplied by the laboratory.

Coating manufacturers supply product information literature that should be studied for updates.

Chapter 9

PRESCRIBING ABSORPTIVE LENSES

INTRODUCTION

Absorptive lenses are designed either to prevent certain wavelengths from entering the eye or to reduce the intensity of those wavelengths that do enter. While even in 350 B.C. absorptive lenses were known to help patients with acute needs—such as glassblowers exposed to excessive UV and IR radiation—the comfort afforded when visible light of high intensities is absorbed is a relatively recent realization. This understanding is largely the result of research making available lens tints that provide adequate protection for every need. Further enhancement of the role of absorptive lenses resulted from the involvement of styling experts who consistently promote sunwear as desirable fashion accessories that add interest and intrigue to face and costume which continues to this day.

PROPERTIES OF RADIANT ENERGY

Light is a form of radiant energy, electromagnetic in nature and described by specific wavelengths. The wavelengths of radiant energy extend from the shortest cosmic waves, 10^{-14}m in length, to the longest power-transmission wavelengths at 10^8m.

Of these, only the range from 380 to 780nm (where 1nm = 10^{-9}m) can be perceived by the human eye. This is called the *visible spectrum,* or *light,* where the visual system interprets the individual wavelengths as colors. However, the practitioner is concerned not only with the visible spectrum but also with the wavelengths extending slightly to each side.

The UV rays are in the continuation of the visible spectrum at the blue end and consist of UVA from 315 to 400nm, UVB from 280 to 315nm, and UVC from 100 to 280nm. The IR radiations are off the red end of the visible spectrum and are described as near IR from 700 to 1400nm, intermediate IR from 1400 to 5000nm, and far IR from 5000 to 1,000,000nm. Overexposure to these rays can result in ocular discomfort and pathological involvement of the eye and its adnexa.

UVA and UVB rays are found in sunlight; UVC radiation is filtered from sunlight by the earth's atmosphere, especially the ozone layer. Human overexposure to UV radiation is most likely at high altitudes, where the atmosphere is thin, and in the sunlight reflected from any shimmery area such as snow or water. Overexposure is also possible from man-made sources, such as the arcs created during electric welding, and the UV lamps used for a variety of purposes from germicidal applications to pleasurable tanning. Prolonged overexposure to UV rays can result in inflammation of the cornea and the conjunctiva, cancers of the eye and its adnexa, cataracts, pterygia, and retinal disease, to name a few of the implicated disorders.

IR rays can be hazardous, too. Looking directly at sources that produce radiation—direct sunlight, molten substances such as glass and metal, arc lamps, and IR lamps—can result in clouding of the crystalline lens and/or lesions of the retina and choroid if the radiations are of sufficient intensity and duration.

Exposure to the visible spectrum, 380 to 760nm, does not normally lead to pathological disorders. However, individuals who are sensitive to light rays found in normal illumination may experience symptoms described as eyestrain and eye fatigue, and overexposure to the short wavelength (blue) part of the visible spectrum is suspected to contribute to certain retinal dysfunctions.

CLASSIFICATION OF CONVENTIONAL TINTS FOR GLASS LENSES

Clear crown glass lenses transmit 90% to 92% of the radiation between 300nm and 4000nm. These lenses absorb almost

100% of the radiations below 300nm, the short UV rays. Since these absorptions are not always suitable for a specific application, some manufacturers produce a variety of tinted glass lenses. Certain chemicals are added in the ingredients of clear glass during the manufacturing process to result in both a color change and transmission characteristics. The color of the lens, however, does not necessarily indicate its absorptive properties. Two pink lenses, appearing the same shade, for instance, may have different transmission curves. The lens color depends on its absorptive value for the visible spectrum only and even then only determines its general effect upon the light rays. A lens, for example, that absorbs the red, green, and yellow wavelengths more than the blue will appear blue.

The addition of cerium oxide also makes a lens more opaque to UV radiation; if ferrous oxide is added, the lens is more opaque to IR radiation.

Conventional tinted glass lenses are distributed under various trade names, but they can be grouped into one of the following four classifications. The lightest tint in any group is designated by the lowest number or by the letter closest to the beginning of the alphabet.

Note: It is important to note that in the last decade there have been many changes in the availability of tinted glass lenses. Major lens companies have either merged or have discontinued production of all but the most profitable. Vision-Ease Lens remains the major manufacturer of glass lenses in the United States, and for update availability, the company can be queried.

1. **Lenses that evenly reduce the transmission of the visible spectrum while absorbing UV and IR rays.** These lenses can be light enough for indoor wear or dark enough to be classified as sunlenses. The lighter shades are pink and generally designed to transmit 80% to 88% of the visible spectrum. They can be recommended to patients who complain of indoor glare. These individuals usually have light skin and/or large pupils, or may have a psychological need for such a tint. The deeper pinks can be prescribed to albinos for indoor wear (lack of pigment makes these individuals extremely sensitive to light), but it is best to remember that almost always plastic lenses are preferred to glass.

    The most recognizable name for pink tints is Softlite. While Bausch & Lomb, the original manufacturer, has discontinued production, Softlite is such a recognizable name, it may be used to identify certain pink tints on plastic lenses.

Vision-Ease Lens simply uses the actual color; pink 1 and pink 2.

The suntints in this category are gray and offer the finest protection because they absorb harmful UV and IR radiation without distorting the visible spectrum.

The most recognizable is Rayban G15 by Bausch & Lomb (transmission is 15% as it is deep gray in color). As of 1999, Bausch & Lomb sold the prestigious Rayban line to Luxottica.

Vision-Ease Lens, the largest manufacturer of gray sunlenses simply identifies the color as gray 2 (medium gray) and gray 3 (dark gray). Gray 2 has light transmission of 30%; gray 3, 15%.

The choice of a medium-gray or dark-gray tint depends on the patient's subjective reaction to bright illumination. If symptoms are acute, it is best to prescribe the deeper shade. Fashion trends usually set by theatrical personalities also play a role because patients tend to request the color they see on the screen.

2. **Lens tints that absorb UV radiation and transmit the visible spectrum evenly.** The pink tints in this category are satisfactory for patients needing an overall reduction of light transmission. They often complain about general glare, tend to be light complexioned, and have light eyes and/or large pupils.

    The original Cruxite AX, visible light transmission about 83%, was distributed by American Optical Corp. Glass lenses in this category are rarely used today, but the name Cruxite may remain as identification for some pink-tinted plastic lenses.

3. **Lenses that absorb UV and IR rays but show some selectivity for the visible spectrum.** The original general-purpose lens used in this category, manufactured by Therminon Lens Co. and distributed with the trade name Therminon, is available from Vision-Ease under the name Unisol.

Pale greenish-blue in appearance, it is designated for patients needing a slight reduction in the amount of light that enters the eye. However, unless there is a specific reason for its use, the pink tints that have the same reduction in transmission and do not show selectivity in the visible spectrum are a better choice. In addition, many patients find the "Coke bottle" look of the lens a cosmetic detraction. Chances are high that Unisol will be discontinued in the near future.

There are two suntints in this category. One is green in appearance; the other, brown (tan). They are selective in their transmission of the visible spectrum and alter color values slightly. (The gray tints are almost always preferable for sunglasses because they absorb harmful radiation without affecting the visible spectrum.) A green 3 (deep color) is available from Vision-Ease Lens, but basically, other green tints in prescription lenses have been phased out in the United States.

The tan 3 (deep brownish shade) glass lens, index 1.523, available from Vision-Ease, is an excellent absorber of UV and IR rays. The color tends to limit its use to those desiring a cosmetic effect because there is slight distortion in the visible spectrum. Colors are not always seen as "true."

The tan 3 is made in single vision and a number of fused multifocals, including straight-top 25, ST 28, round-top 22 and RT 25, and straight-top trifocals 7 × 25 and 7 × 28mm.

Note: Tan 1 and 2 listed in previous catalogues have been discontinued.

4. **Tints designed for special uses.** The lenses in this category are highly selective in their absorptive properties. Since each tint is drastically different from any other, they are classified according to color with an explanation of their use.

   a. Rose didymium filter. This lens has a unique filter designed to be used by glass blowers. It greatly reduces transmission while absorbing harmful UV and IR radiation. It is a standard order in single vision and a flat-top 25mm bifocal.

Vision-Ease will custom make an FT 28mm bifocal and a few trifocal designs. Query the laboratory for specifics.

Note: This lens is not recommended for welders. Excel manufacturers a green welding lens in plano. It is not available in prescription form.

b. Thindex (high index glass). High index glass is designed to reduce thickness and weight compared with crown glass (index 1.523). Thindex is manufactured in three different indices: 1.60, 1.70, and 1.80. In 1.60 and 1.80 indices, only single-vision prescriptions are available. The 1.70 index lens is also made in flat-top 25mm and FT 28mm bifocals. There is considerable chromatic aberration through the segments, so Thindex may not be a good choice for many patients.

c. X-Ray, index 1.80. This lens, available from Vision-Ease, provides protection from x-ray radiation. It cannot be strengthened to meet the U.S. Food and Drug Administration (FDA) ruling for "safety." Therefore, a patient must sign an impact-resistance waiver, or the practitioner can order Corlon polyurethane applied to the back surface. This then allows the lens to comply with the impact-resistance laws.

d. Yellow-tinted lenses. Often referred to as "shooting" lenses, these tints absorb most of the UV rays but have a high transmission for IR rays. They transmit the visible spectrum by about 70%. Theoretically, the tint "cuts" through early-morning haze to render distant objects more visible. However, scientific studies often concluded that this claim was not valid. Scored marksmanship tests taken with individuals wearing the yellow lens were compared with scores when the lenses were not worn. The majority of the marksmen did not score higher wearing yellow-tinted lenses. However, this is a controversial subject. Patients often comment that wearing "shooting glasses" during cloudy or foggy hours improves their marksmanship, and others claim the glasses make skiing easier during the twilight hours. This reaction is a possibility because the yellow lens has the ability to filter blue light, the shortest-wavelength light in the spectrum. (The blue can focus in front of the retina resulting in a blurred image on the retina.)

While still available in plano form, particularly in sporting goods stores, these lenses have been discontinued in prescription form.

e. Extra–dark green lenses. Visibility is considerably reduced when these lenses are worn since light transmission is a very low 5% to 10%. Distributed in plano lenses for use by welders, etc., for specific industrial wear, they are available primarily from Excel.

f. Dark smoke lenses. These lenses (when available) were grayish-black in appearance. Since they reduced visibility markedly, they were used only for temporary relief of acute photophobia resulting from a pathological condition. In professional offices throughout the United States, dark smoked-glass lenses have been replaced by plastic designs (no prescription) in cardboard frames as a precaution against transmitting eye infections.

POLAROID GLASS LENSES

Perhaps the greatest advance in the field of lens design within the past decade is the improvement of Polaroid lenses and their availability in a great number of designs and prescriptions. No longer limited to laminated crown glass, Polaroids are also available in single-vision high-index, 1.56, plastic CR 39 and plastic polycarbonates. This welcomed expansion means that many more patients can enjoy the advantages of wearing Polaroid lenses. This section deals primarily with glass Polaroid lenses. Other designs are discussed later in this chapter.

All polarized lenses are designed to eliminate glare reflected from flat surfaces at certain angles. The original Polaroids were fashioned from films of polarizing material laminated between clear or lightly tinted glass lenses. The polarizing material consists of nitrocellulose packed with ultramicroscopic crystals of herapathite having their optic axes parallel to one another. Most polarized filters transmitted about 37% of incident light. All quality Polaroid sunlenses function in an excellent manner to reduce glare from "shiny" horizontal surfaces, such as sunlight on light-colored highways, water, and snow.

For many years, Polaroid lenses were manufactured in glass only and available exclusively through American Optical Corp. (now American Optical Lens Company). Later a polarized lens was distributed by Liberty Optical Co. under the trade name Vergopol. These lenses had limited tint and prescription availability.

Melibrand then introduced a lens under the trade name Polar-ray, which is still available. It is manufactured in single vision with a number of color choices; gray A and C and brown C. There is also a medium gray B shade with a mirrored front surface.

The drawback with the original Polaroid lenses that made eye care professionals hesitate to prescribe them was the basic construction. The two glass lenses had a polarizing film laminated with adhesive to either side of the polarizing film. Eventually, the lenses would separate from the film making them useless to the wearer.

In the early 1990s, manufacturers found a way to suspend the polarized film within the lens mold. Thus, the polarizing film became an integral part of the lenses (no adhesives were necessary), and as production methods improved (called *molecular bonding*), delamination no longer existed. Today every polarized lens is guaranteed by the manufacturer against separation.

There is a wide choice in prescription glass lenses. The popular bifocal and trifocal designs available include straight-top (flat-top) 28mm and 35mm bifocals; ST 7 × 25 and ST 7 × 28mm trifocals in gray C, the deeper gray 3 tint. Lighter shades of gray (1 and 2) are made in single vision. There is a limited prescription choice in brown, yellow, and amber. There are also mirrored single-vision lenses in some tints. A high-index glass lens, 1.56, is available in single vision in gray C and brown C.

With the wide expansion of availability in Polaroid lenses, it is always best to query the local laboratory for updates if other than a standard lens style or color is desired.

POLAROID PLASTIC LENSES

Plano and single-vision prescription lenses are available from many manufacturers and include CR 39 plastic, high-index

1.56 and polycarbonates. The CR 39 designs are also available in flat-top 28mm and flat-top 35mm bifocals. There are flat-top 7 × 28 and flat-top 8 × 35 trifocals. Some plastic progressive addition lenses in Polaroid have become available, and the local laboratory can be queried for updates.

Corning released a plastic photochromic lens design in early 2000 called Sun Sensor. The high index of refraction is 1.56. The photochromic material throughout the lens allows it to change uniform color in 60 seconds. Manufactured in a gray tint that varies from 86% transmission indoors to 17% in its darkest stage (color change comfortable for most patients), it is available in single vision, FT 28 and FT 35 bifocals, and a flat-top 7 × 28mm trifocal.

The Nupolar polarized lenses released in the latter 1990s by Younger Optics has the polarizing film in the lens itself. Encasing the film makes the lens less likely to be affected by atmospheric conditions and therefore able to retain the absorptive properties for a longer period of time.

The lens is manufactured in CR 39 plastic and in polycarbonate plastic. The CR 39 is available in a range of −8.00D to +6.00D in single-vision lenses and in flat-top 28, FT 35mm bifocals and a flat-top 7 × 28mm trifocal. Currently the single-vision series is made in gray 1, gray 3, and brown C. The same colors are available in the FT 28mm bifocal. The FT 35 and FT 7 × 28 trifocal are made are the deep gray 3 only, but the tint availability may be expanded soon.

Younger Optics promotes the light gray 1 as a tint over which custom colors can be applied. Antireflection coatings will also adhere; so will a mirror coating for a fashion effect if that is desired.

The Nupolar polarized lens has been released in the Image progressive addition design (see Chapter 5, "Prescribing 'Invisible' Multifocals") in the deep shades of gray 3 and brown 3. The color range may be expanded in the future.

Polycarbonate Polaroids are manufactured in single vision, gray 3 only. Additions may be made in the future.

There are advantages to wearing Polaroid lenses. They are as follows:

1.   **Reduction of surface glare improves visibility.** Glare adversely effects visibility, and for driving, this can be especially hazardous. Those who drive long hours on freeway roads, such as truck drivers and bus drivers, are particularly vulnerable. Surface glare

from water is especially annoying to water skiers, boaters, fishermen, and anyone who works on or near bodies of water. Surface glare from snow is also a major problem, particularly for skiers and anyone controlling a sledding device.

2. **Polarized lenses as protection.** All Polaroid lenses protect the eyes from both direct and reflected UV rays. UV radiation can cause snow blindness and also contribute to early age-related cataracts, pterygium, and cancer of the skin around the eye area.

PHOTOCHROMIC GLASS LENSES

Photochromics, promoted as light-sensitive sunsensor lenses, are designed to darken when exposed to UV radiation. The color change is achieved by the addition of silver halide crystals evenly dispersed in the glass. Each is about 1/100,000mm in diameter, tightly packed so as to avoid scattering of visible light.

There are a number of photochromic glass designs widely advertised to the profession and to the public. Most are manufactured by Corning, Inc. (formerly Corning Glass Works) and sold to optical companies, each of whom then distributes them under an individual label. Before discussing the characteristics of each design, fundamentals applicable to all are presented. These need to be understood for recommendation purposes:

1. Photochromic lenses darken only when exposed to UV rays. If these rays are blocked (for instance, behind the windshield of a car), the lenses remain in the lightened stage. Conversely, the lenses may darken on a dull day when UV rays are in the atmosphere or indoors under UV lights.

2. Photochromic glass lenses need to go through as many as ten light-to-dark cycles before they darken to their potential.

3. If photochromic lenses are not worn for a period of time, usually exceeding a month, the light-to-dark cycles have to be repeated. The darkening performance never deteriorates, however, and can be reactivated indefinitely.

4. Photochromic lenses may darken but not to their maximum on a foggy or misty day.

5. The color change in photochromic lenses is affected by the temperature; the colder the day, the darker they will become. Some may reach a different maximum color on cold days.

6. The prescription must be close to the same for both eyes. If the right lens, for instance, is $+3.00 - 1.00 \times 90$ and the left a $+6.00D$ sphere, the lenses will not darken evenly.

7. Photochromic glass lenses are usually thicker than conventional lenses. While density is 2.54g/ml and index is 1.523, the same as standard crown glass, additional weight theoretically should not be a problem. However, the thicker the lens, the darker it will become for a given sunlight exposure. Therefore, local laboratories insist upon determining the thickness.

8. The color change in photochromic glass lenses may be altered in an unpredictable fashion if lens coatings are used. The lens may stay in a darkened stage when the wearer returns indoors or may darken to a color foreign to the design.

9. All photochromics of a specific model do not lighten and darken in an absolute pattern. Batches produced one month can and will vary from those manufactured at a later date. Photochromic lenses should therefore be ordered in pairs.

10. While photochromic designs absorb UV radiation, they all transmit IR radiation. If a patient is exposed excessively or continuously to direct or reflected sunlight, to molten glass or molten metal, then glass lenses such as Rayban G15 that absorb IR as well as UV rays need to be prescribed.

11. Photochromic lenses should be chemically tempered to make them impact resistant. Heat treating lowers the transmission and, as with all lenses processed in this manner, makes them more susceptible to spontaneous breakage. There also can be slight surface defacement when lenses are heat treated (see Chapter 10, "Impact-Resistant [Safety] Lenses").

SPECIFIC PHOTOCHROMIC DESIGNS

Historic Overview

To understand the progress of glass photochromic designs, a historic overview is in order. The following are no longer available and it is not likely the practitioner will still see patients wearing the lenses.

1. Photogray Lenses (No Longer Available). These were the first photochromic lenses and were introduced in 1968. In the palest stage, light transmission was 83%. When darkened to their maximum 44% transmission, the medium gray color was not dark enough in bright sunlight for most patients.

2. Photosun Lenses (No Longer Available). The next photochromics to be introduced were Photosun lenses. The Photosun designs were light gray indoors with 65% light transmission. In the maximum darkness stage, the lens became a dark gray having 20% light transmission. Because it remained relatively dark indoors, the lens had limited use and was soon discontinued.

3. Photobrown Lenses (No Longer Available). These lenses were promoted as clear indoors with an average light transmission of 88%. There was a pale residual yellowish-green tint that was not attractive. Maximum darkness appeared to be about 60%. The lenses did not darken sufficiently in bright sunlight, and the design was soon discontinued. Very few of these lenses were ever prescribed.

4. Fused Light and Dark Photochromics (No Longer Available). These original multifocal lenses became available in 1975 and were a welcome addition for the presbyopic patient. Today, the improved designs of fused multifocals are usually prescribed in Photogray Extra (described later in this chapter).

5. Sun Magic Photochromics (Discontinued). These lenses were manufactured by Schott Optical Glass. They differed from other photochromics in that less time was needed for fading after the darkening stage had taken place. They were available only in plano and single-vision corrections in a wide variety of colors that included gray, brown, tan, green, and blue. They are no longer manufactured, but Schott does continue to make unusual colors for certain prescriptions. The local laboratory can be queried for specifics.

CURRENTLY PRESCRIBED PHOTOCHROMIC GLASS LENSES

Note: The percentage of transmission given for each lens varies slightly depending on lens thickness, temperature, and tempering state. At one time, all given transmission curves were based on lens exposure to natural sunlight at 25°C (77°F) in plano form 2mm thick. Newer texts give measurements conducted within a temperature range of 72°F to 78°F (22°C to 26°C), so it is possible that released fade/dark percentages will vary slightly from those given in this chapter. It is especially important to remember when prescribing current photochromic glass designs that the released transmission curves be for plano lenses 2mm thick.

1. Photogray Extra. This is the most popular photochromic lens and is distributed by all major glass manufacturers. In its lightest stage, the tint allows 85% transmission. At its darkest stage, which is achieved in bright sunshine, the color becomes a deep gray with 22% transmission (Figure 9.1).

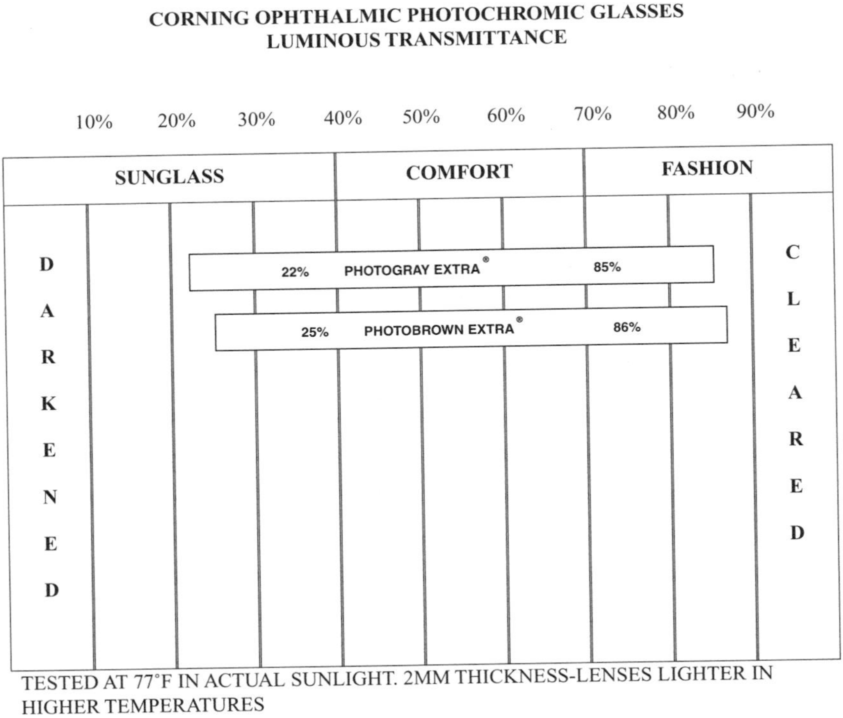

CORNING OPHTHALMIC PHOTOCHROMIC GLASSES
LUMINOUS TRANSMITTANCE

TESTED AT 77°F IN ACTUAL SUNLIGHT. 2MM THICKNESS-LENSES LIGHTER IN HIGHER TEMPERATURES

FIGURE 9.1 *Photogray Extra*

The change from light to dark takes place in about 60 seconds, which is quicker than with previous photochromics. Photogray Extra is available in almost any desired design, including single-vision, and all popular fused, flat-top (straight-top) multifocals; FT25mm, FT28mm, and FT35mm bifocals; FT7 × 25 and FT7 × 28mm trifocals and double-segment occupational designs. In the fused designs, the segment glass is clear, so the near/intermediate areas remain in a lighter shade when the lens darkens. Photogray Extra lenses are also manufactured in one-piece, Executive-style bifocals, seamless/blended bifocals, and a great number of progressive-addition lens designs. Querying the local laboratory for updates is in order.

2. Photobrown Extra. This lens is a deep brown color in the darkest stage and has 25% light transmission. In the faded stage, it has 86% transmission. The design is not as widely prescribed as the Photogray Extra, so it is best to query the local laboratory for current availability of multifocal styles. In the fused designs, the segment areas are lighter than the distance when the lens is exposed to bright illumination.

3. Photosun II. Photosun II is designed for use as a sunlens in both the faded and darkened stages. The lens is a gray color and when lightened becomes a medium gray with 40% light transmission. In the darkest stage it transmits 12% of the visible light. Photosun II is not for the patient having only one pair of glasses. The color in the faded stage is too dark indoors and is dangerous for night driving. Chances are high this lens will soon be discontinued. Many patients find it too deep for comfort in the darkest stage and that it adversely affects visual acuity. The local laboratory needs to be queried for availability of multifocal designs.

4. Custom Photochromic Lenses. Corning can produce any color with desired absorption curves and makes specific lenses as exclusives to optical companies upon request. The lenses can be solid or feature gradient colors. However, custom photochromics are expensive and therefore relatively rare.

5. Corning Photochromic Filter Lenses. The Corning Photochromic Filter (CPF) series are lenses distributed by Corning Medical Optics for wear by low-vision patients. Three designs were originally released: CPF 511, CPF 527, and CPF 550. These lenses absorb UV radiation as well as the blue end

of the visible spectrum. The three digits refer to the wavelength in nanometers to which the lenses attenuate.

CPF lenses have a very distinctive color range. Depending on the design, they vary from red to yellow-amber. Like all photochromics, the lenses fade in low illumination and darken in bright sunlight. Specifically designed to cut acute glare that adversely affects the partially sighted, CPF lenses are considered a major breakthrough, since certain pathological conditions result in a glare factor that limits visibility.

The CPF 511 lens has 16% light transmission in the darkened stage, with a resultant deep orange-yellow color. The lightened stage is a yellow-amber tone exhibiting 47% transmission. The CPF 511 is recommended for patients with immature cataracts, diabetic retinopathy, and for aphakes who have not had a lens implant.

CPF 527 has 12% transmission in the darkest stage and 37% in the lightest. Both stages are deep tones, with the lighter being an orange-amber color. CPF 527 is recommended for patients with severe photophobia regardless of cause.

The CPF 550 is a very dark lens, 5% transmission in the darkened stage (seriously affecting the vision of a normally sighted person) becoming a reddish-amber in the lightened stage with 21% transmission. CPF 550 lenses are designed for patients with retinitis pigmentosa.

Before prescribing the CPF series, the practitioner should be study carefully the literature prepared by Corning Medical Optics. Each lens has transmission properties making it best (or suitable) for patients with certain vision problems and/or pathological conditions.

CPF lenses are available in plano form as well as prescription single-vision, bifocal, trifocal, and lenticular designs. Only certain optical laboratories can finish the prescription lenses, so inquiry about ordering procedures is critical. Information regarding the CPF series is available by contacting Corning, Inc., 1-800-742-5273.

PLASTIC PHOTOCHROMICS

Transitions Photochromics

Never in the history of tinted lenses has there been as much advertising to the public, primarily via television, as for the series of photochromic plastic lenses called Transitions (available through a great number of distributors).

These lenses lighten and darken according to a chemical reaction of sunlight on the front surface of the lens, which is imbedded with a thin layer of an organic material (indolino spironaphthoxzine). The tints most advertised to the eyecare professional remain a hint of color in the faded stage; in the darkest stage, the color is equivalent to a suntint.

These are the available designs:

1. Transitions III Gray and Transitions III Brown. These lenses are made of a CR 39 type plastic having a 1.50 index of refraction. Basically, transmission is the same for both—only the color is different. They fade to 87% transmission, which is a bare tinge of color, and darken to 22% transmission (a deep suntint color). Both are available in single vision, flat-top 28 and FT 35mm bifocals, FT 7 × 28 and FT 8 × 35mm trifocals. Some progressive addition designs are also available. Querying the local laboratory is in order.

2. Transitions XTRActive. This is a CR 39 type plastic, index 1.5. These lenses become very dark in full sunlight, with 11% transmission (thus the term XTRActive). Indoors there is a noticeable residual color. The range of multifocal availability is the same as Transitions III previously described.

3. Transitions III High Index. This lens is available in both 1.54 and 1.55 index in gray or brown. Basically, light transmission is comparable with that with an index of 1.50 (described earlier). There is limited multifocal availability, so the local laboratory should be queried for updates.

4. Transitions III Polycarbonate. This lens is the thinnest available design in Transitions. In its lightest stage there is a slight blush cast (unlike the other Transitions III designs). In full sunlight, it does not darken as much as Transitions CR 39 type plastic. There is a very limited multifocal availability.

Note: The original Transitions Plus, which faded to 84% indoor transmission and 28% transmission in full sunlight, has been discontinued.

There are some drawbacks to all plastic photochromic lenses. Over time, the color change process gradually deteriorates, but by then the patient may need a new prescription. While all Transitions lenses come with a Scratch Guard coating, if an antireflection coating is applied, performance is reduced by about 15%. It possibly could be placed on the back surface when it is necessary to reduce overhead and back glare that may be annoying to the patient.

The decision to prescribe Transitions plastic photochromics over glass photochromic lenses (both absorb all harmful UV rays) depends on the patient's request and the practitioner's professional judgment. Glass photochromics are heavier but have a stable light-to-dark color change (discussed earlier in this chapter). Transitions, being lighter, are much more comfortable, an important factor for many patients.

Note: Photolites, the original plastic photochromic lenses introduced in the late 1980s by American Optical Corp., and designed primarily as fashion tints, have long been discontinued. They did not darken sufficiently for use as sunlenses. In bright sunlight Photolites became a light blue color that faded after prolonged exposure to UV radiation. The 90% to 92% indoor transmission was comparable with that of a clear lens. It is not likely that patients would still be wearing these lenses.

Hard-Resin CR 39 (Plastic) Absorptive Lenses

Tints in any desired shade are easily obtained by dyeing a plastic CR 39 lens. Popular fashion hues are the soft pinks and blues, dove gray, and pale tan. If light transmission is 80% to 85%, these colors do not abnormally distort the visible spectrum.

Absorptive curves for plastic lenses are rarely if ever made available, but if the fashion shades are vivid, natural colors will appear distorted or drastically altered. Patients must be discouraged from wearing such deep tones when driving a car, operating a motorcycle, or flying a plane, because the change in color perception could result in a misinterpretation of important signals (e.g., red and green lights). These tints are especially dangerous if worn at night and/or in combination with tinted windshields. Unfortunately, celebrities sometimes wear "weird" colors such as purple, red, or orange lens hues, so younger patients may request them.

Initially, the use of hard coatings to make the surfaces of CR 39 lenses scratch resistant resulted in an inability to tint such lenses properly. For the most part, these problems have been solved.

Polycarbonate Plastic Absorptive Lenses

All polycarbonate lenses, even when clear, absorb all harmful UV radiation. The addition of color creates a fashion look and/or results in tints deep enough for use out-of-doors. Polycarbonate lenses have hard coatings on both surfaces, so at one time obtaining deeper shades for sunwear was a problem. However, this problem rarely exists today. Absorptive curves for tinted polycarbonate lenses are seldom, if ever, made available.

COLOR COATINGS FOR GLASS LENSES

Absorptive curves for color coatings applied to glass lenses are almost always available from the manufacturer. Some absorb IR as well as UV rays. In most cases the practitioner can prescribe them knowing their effects on the various wavelengths. The lens coatings that are vivid in color for a fashion effect have the same dangers as the bright plastic tints. The hues that are very pale and appear to be just a "cast" of color have a light transmission of about 88% to 90% and in most cases are as safe to wear as clear lenses.

EFFECT OF PRESCRIPTION ON LENS COLOR

Color is uniform in a tinted glass lens (an oxide is added to the ingredients of clear glass) only when center and edge thicknesses are equal (plano). Pale tinted glass lenses rarely present a problem, but when prescription lenses are deep in intensity, the problem of maintaining uniform color can be critical.

A convex lens, being thicker in the center, has a deeper color in that area. With a concave correction, the reverse is true: the center, which is thinner than the edges, will be a lighter shade. A cylindrical correction can appear to have a darker or lighter band of color, depending on the prescription.

When the correction involved is less than plus or minus 2.00D, the difference in a deeper color is not obvious enough to present a problem. In a lens correction ±2.25D to ±4.00D, usually the color difference can be minimized effectively by requesting the laboratory to control thickness (i.e., to keep the center of minus lenses thicker than conventional lenses). A frame can be dispensed that limits the horizontal box measurement of the lens to 50mm to 52mm. The larger the lens, the more obvious is the color variation.

When the correction is greater than ±4.00D, or if it varies greatly between the two eyes (e.g., +1.00D for the right eye and −3.00D for the left eye), it is always necessary to use some method of tinting that results in uniform color. There are two possibilities. One involves dying a plastic lens; the other is applying a color coating to the glass lens.

The tint of a plastic lens is impregnated into the lens surface, making it uniform regardless of the correction. However, several precautions are necessary when prescribing plastic sunlenses. While they satisfactorily cut down general illumination and eliminate harmful UV rays, they do not absorb IR light. If the patient is exposed continuously to IR radiation (e.g., a glass-blower or an outdoor worker in the desert), it is necessary to prescribe a lens having known absorptive properties.

Care of plastic CR 39 lenses can be more involved than that of those fashioned of glass, and this may be an inconvenience when sunwear is involved. To maintain a scratch-free surface, dust must be washed off before the lens is wiped clean. Silicone papers cannot be used, because they mar the lenses. On the other hand, the added safety of plastic lenses is often an important consideration, particularly when worn while operating a motor vehicle.

Note: If the lens surface has a scratch-resistant coating, it can be cleaned by any conventional method. However, it must be remembered that this coating may be only on the front surface, and caution is necessary so as not to scratch the back surface.

Uniform color can also be obtained by applying a color coating to a clear glass lens. The lens is cut to the required size and shape before the coating process takes place. This makes it possible to prescribe large sunlenses that offer maximum protection. Absorption curves of color coatings are available, allowing the practitioner to prescribe them when absorption properties are critical to the patient's needs.

There are a few disadvantages that have to be considered when prescribing color-coated glass lenses. The coating may have a "metallic" look, although this problem is greatly lessened when the color is applied by a quality laboratory. Another disadvantage may be that coated lenses need to be cleaned frequently. They attract dust that adheres to the lens surface. To be cleaned properly, they should be run under warm water before wiping. The problem is minimized with a permanent clear coating on *both* surfaces designed to allow silicone papers to be used for cleaning.

The weight of the glass may also be a problem, especially if the lenses are oversize. Whenever possible, it is best to recommend plastic lenses.

AVAILABILITY OF TINTED LENS PRESCRIPTIONS

A drastic change has taken place in the manufacture and stocking of glass absorptive lenses. Since tinted hard-resin lens are prescribed with increasing frequency, glass lenses that have an oxide added in the manufacturing process are no longer readily available in various powers. It is highly unlikely that a wide selection of colors is stocked at a local laboratory. However, major manufacturers can supply conventional tints in single vision, bifocals, and trifocals to a local laboratory, often on an overnight basis so this is rarely a limitation.

A good possibility is color coating a prescription clear lens. Every coating company distributes kits featuring sample colors that are easily duplicated.

The popular Photogray Extra in a wide range of prescriptions and multifocal designs may be stocked at a local laboratory. Other standard photochromic prescription glass lenses are available within a short waiting period from the manufacturer (usually Vision-Ease).

SUNFRAME FASHIONS

Every major sunwear manufacturer introduces a new line of sunfashions twice a year and many as often as four times a year. These designs create a specific type of fashion value and utilize tinted plano lenses. If given to the patient in this form, absorptive properties must be ascertained because the "color" lenses may not be optical quality. They are in the frame so the eyecare professional and the patient can visualize the finished prescription appearance.

If dark lenses are not mounted into the frame during the initial frame selection, the patient may be disappointed in the cosmetic effect when the sunwear is delivered. Usually the eyewear appears "too small" on the face, an illusion resulting from the darkness of the lenses contrasting with skin tone. Although the smaller effect has become a popular fashion, the patient should be prepared for "the look." For the best protection against the sun's rays, larger eyeframes should be recommended, although patients may prefer more current styles.

Sunwear that curves toward the temples (goggle sunframes) may be worn by skiers and contact lens patients. When objects are viewed through the periphery of a lens mounted into a "curved" frame, distortion is present even in a plano lens. Patients may find this annoying even if the distortion is slight. When a high prescription is involved, the problem can be critical. The higher the correction, the greater is the cylindrical effect that results in distortion (see Chapter 14, "Prescription Changes Induced by Lens Tilt"). It is usually best not to recommend a "goggle" curved-frame design for prescription lenses. However, in corrections up to ±1.00D the distortion may be slight enough that patients can tolerate it, particularly if the angle of the curvature is limited to 10°.

Fit-over frames utilizing tinted plano lenses are cumbersome and can make a poor appearance. The older styles could mar the front surface of prescription lenses. Newer designs hold the fit-overs away from the lenses, but patients should be encouraged to get separate prescription sunwear, which is more comfortable as well as practical.

WHEN TO PRESCRIBE SUNWEAR

All patients benefit from wearing quality tinted lenses (in prescription if necessary) when sunlight is bright or the glare is excessive. It is critical that close to 100% UV absorption be ascertained. Such tints provide a more comfortable outdoor environment and improve visual acuity adversely affected by annoying reflections. They also protect again pathologic conditions of the eye caused by UV rays. For many patients, sunwear is a necessity. Most contact lens wearers, for instance, are rarely comfortable out-of-doors without adequate protection against the sun's rays. (The eyewear also protects against the dust and dirt that can fly under the contact lenses.)

The gray tints in glass lenses that absorb UV and IR radiation without altering the visible spectrum offer the finest complete sunwear protection. The shade prescribed depends upon subjective symptoms. If the patient reports mild annoyance in bright illumination, the medium gray tint is usually the best choice.

Since in actuality most patients need only UV-absorbing lenses, quality CR 39 plastic, polycarbonates, and the photochromic designs offer proper protection in prescription lenses. (Plano plastic lenses are easily available with IR absorbers but unfortunately not in prescription form.)

In light of the fact that the ozone layer, which protects the earth against UV radiation is being depleted, all patients who are in the sun even for short periods of time should wear UV protective lenses. UV radiation can cause early cataract formation as well as malignant disease of the skin and tissues of the eye areas. If the eyewear is purchased "over-the-counter," it is critical to read the label to insure 95% to 100% protection against UV. The actual color is not a guideline. A gray lens, for example, may only alter the visible spectrum and have no effect on harmful UV radiation.

Chapter 10

IMPACT-RESISTANT (SAFETY) LENSES

INTRODUCTION

A policy statement issued by the U.S. Food and Drug Administration (FDA) made it illegal not to prescribe impact-resistant lenses as of January 1, 1972. If the practitioner decides for a specific case not to prescribe them, certain conditions need to be followed. These are stated under section (c) of the law and are quoted in this chapter.

The essentials of the law—those factors particularly pertinent to the practitioner—are noted in this introduction. However, changes are possible, and it is the practitioner's responsibility to know the legal aspects affecting the eyecare professions. Any additional information desired may be obtained by querying the federal government. Local laboratories also can be queried, because they are knowledgeable about all changes. As of January 1, 1972, the following ruling regarding impact-resistant lenses became law.

Title 21—Food and Drugs
Chapter 1—Food and Drug Administration
Department of Health, Education, and Welfare
Subchapter A—General

Part 3—statements of general policy or interpretation
Use of Impact-Resistant Lenses in Eyeglasses and Sunglasses. . . .

(a) Examination of data available on the frequency of eye injuries resulting from the shattering of ordinary crown glass lenses indicate that the use of such lenses constitutes an avoidable hazard to the eye of the wearer.

(b) The consensus of the ophthalmic community is that the number of eye injuries would be substantially reduced by the use in eyeglasses and sunglasses of either plastic lenses, heat-treated crown glass lenses, or lenses made impact-resistant by other methods.

(c) To protect the public more adequately from potential eye injury, eyeglasses and sunglasses must be fitted with impact-resistant lenses, except in those cases where the physician or optometrist finds that such lenses will not fulfill the visual requirements of the particular patient, directs in writing the use of other lenses, and gives written notification thereof to the patient.

(d) The physician or optometrist shall have the option of ordering heat-treated glass lenses, plastic lenses, laminated glass lenses or glass lenses made impact-resistant by other methods; however, all such lenses must be capable of withstanding an impact test in which a $5/8$ inch steel ball weighing approximately 0.56 ounce is dropped from a height of 50 inches upon the horizontal upper surface of the lens. . . .

Lenses classified as impact resistant and often referred to as safety lenses have been available for many years. However, until the above policy statement by the FDA made it illegal not to prescribe impact-resistant lenses, these lenses were recommended at the discretion of the practitioner. Now in the prescribing of non−impact-resistant lenses, certain conditions must be followed; they are stated under section (c). As a result, almost all lenses used in the United States are manufactured of an impact-resistant material or are made impact resistant by certain methods that give them a protective quality. Few eyecare professionals ever apply the exception stated under (c), since it makes them more susceptible to possible legal complications.

The law includes a complete explanation of the method that must be used to test lenses (e.g., where the ball will strike the lens). These specifications are followed by the laboratory that fills the prescription. If the practitioner tempers lenses in the office, detailed information regarding the equipment and related matters can be obtained by querying the federal government. (Not every lens needs to be tested. For example, Executive glass bifocal and trifocal designs whose edges could chip are exempt, as are almost all plastic designs. Further details are available from the FDA.)

Until the law became effective, the term *safety lenses* was used synonymously with *impact-resistant lenses.* However, patient confusion—most lay persons interpret *safety* as meaning an unbreakable lens—has resulted in a recommendation by the American Optometric Association that the term *safety lenses* be eliminated. Instead, an explanation should be offered the patient that although impact-resistant lenses are designed to withstand considerable pressure, any lens can and will break if struck with enough force (the possible exception being polycarbonate lenses, which may crack under certain conditions but will not break into splinters).

TYPES OF IMPACT-RESISTANT LENSES

Lenses classified as impact resistant are available in a number of forms. The best are manufactured from CR 39 hard resin or polycarbonate. Others are made of optical-quality glass modified to give a protective quality. Impact-resistant lenses made of glass are further subdivided into chemically tempered, heat-treated (sometimes called *air-treated*), and laminated lenses.

Polycarbonate Lenses and Plastic (CR 39 Hard Resin) Lenses

There are many ramifications involving plastic lenses, particularly the tremendous strides made in the design of both single-vision and multifocal lenses. Chapter 7, "Plastic Ophthalmic Lenses," is devoted exclusively to this subject. This chapter concerns itself with the advantages from a safety viewpoint.

Polycarbonate lenses are advertised as virtually unbreakable. The same material is used in the manufacture of bullet-proof vests. These designs offer the patient the most protection from potential injury.

CR 39 lenses exhibit a high degree of safety. Research shows that a chemically tempered glass lens appears to withstand the same force as a plastic CR 39, although when it does break, there is a kickback property whereby glass particles can be imbedded into the eye tissue and surrounding facial area. These bits of glass are often difficult to locate and remove, particularly if a clear (transparent) lens breaks. This kickback property was not noted when hard-resin lenses were broken during scientific studies; the pieces were likely to be large rather than splinters and tended to stay contained in the frame.

While all plastic lenses are inherently impact resistant, if the lens is coated (scratch-resistant coatings, antireflection coatings), glass-like coatings can reduce impact resistance. When the newer high-index lenses are ground to 1.5mm or less center thickness (for cosmetic value), most will pass the drop-ball test. If they don't, however, a special primer coating can dissipate some of the impact energy (this coating is placed on all high-index plastic with a 1.00mm center thickness).

Glass Impact-Resistant Lenses

Chemically Tempered Lenses. Chemical strengthening is the best process used to make conventional glass lenses impact resistant. It was developed for ophthalmic use by Corning Glass Works when it became obvious that the FDA ruling might force practitioners to prescribe heat-treated (air-tempered) lenses, which have serious drawbacks, as discussed later in this chapter. Chemical tempering involves a chemical ion exchange between sodium ions in the glass and potassium ions in a specially prepared salt bath. Although introduced over three decades ago, use of chemical tempering had been limited primarily to automobile and aircraft windshields and to laboratory glassware.

There are several advantages to prescribing chemically tempered over heat-treated lenses. Chemically tempered lenses maintain excellent optics without the warpage noted on the surfaces of air-tempered lenses. It is possible to manufacture a chemically tempered lens in a thinner form and still comply with the FDA ruling. Chemically treated lenses in the 1.3mm to 1.5mm minimum thickness range have proved under testing conditions to be stronger than 2.2mm heat-treated lenses.

The chemical strengthening process takes longer than heat treating. Originally, it was recommended that all glass crown lenses be placed for 15 to 16 hours in the molten salt bath. Laboratories usually immerse the edged lenses overnight so they were ready for frame insertion the next day. However, it has been learned that, depending on the method used, the process can be reduced to as low as 4 hours and the lens will still pass the FDA drop-ball test.

The chemical formula of the salt bath for making photochromics impact resistant varies from that of crown lenses. Laboratories therefore have two sets of chemical tempering equipment so that all glass lenses can be treated during the same time period. Most still process the lenses overnight to insure impact resistance.

The possibility of spontaneous breakage, resulting in injuries if the lens "explodes" while the patient is wearing the glasses, is a major problem with heat-treated lenses. While this has not been known to occur with a chemically tempered lens, the tendency exists if it is subjected to deep scratches extending beyond the ion-exchange layer. For this reason Corning Glass Works continues to recommend tempering for 15 to 16 hours, although less time may be needed to produce a lens meeting the FDA regulation.

Unlike heat-treated lenses, those that are chemically strengthened can be resurfaced to make a small prescription change or to remove minor scratches. To make the lenses impact resistant again, reprocessing in the salt bath is required.

If a coated lens is placed in the molten salt bath, the color coating and/or the antireflection coating are removed by the chemical. Coatings have to be applied after tempering has taken place. A tinted lens that owes its color to an oxide added to the ingredients of clear glass can be chemically tempered without affecting its appearance or seriously changing the absorptive properties of the color. (There is a very slight alteration in the IR end of the spectrum.)

Although a verifying certificate accompanies the lenses with the chemical-tempering process, there are few ways to test for the procedure. When viewed under the polariscope, some high plus, chemically tempered lenses exhibit a shape similar to a Maltese cross, but other chemically tempered lenses are free of a distinguishing pattern. This should not pose a problem since optical laboratories keep records for the FDA.

Heat-treated (Air-treated) Lenses. Before the introduction of chemically strengthened ophthalmic lenses, glass lenses were made impact resistant by the heat-treating method. Such lenses exhibited serious drawbacks. Heat tempering consists of heating the glass lens almost to the point of melting and then cooling it quickly by a blast of air—thus the procedure is sometimes called *air tempering.* This causes the surfaces to contract, building up pressures that should make the lens harder and stronger. However, if it is not properly heat treated, or if it is scratched, the lens is less impact resistant than an untreated lens and also becomes prone to what the optical industry refers to as *spontaneous breakage.* In other words, the lens can shatter without an apparent foreign stress. The results can be disastrous if the breakage occurs while the patient is wearing the glasses. This confusion is eloquently described in an article by Barbara Katz that appeared in the *National Observer* some time ago:

> I had been browsing . . . when suddenly I heard a sharp cracking noise, felt something hit my right eye and I screamed. When I gingerly opened my eyes, I found myself staring at a crazy-quilt world. The right lens of my glasses had burst for no apparent reason . . . small splinters dusted my face and some it seemed had entered my right eye.

The American Optometric Association has designed a card imprint, explaining that heat-treated lenses should be replaced if they become scratched. However, a far superior procedure would be the elimination of heat-treated lenses and the prescribing of plastic or chemically tempered lenses. There are no cases on record where either have spontaneously broken on the patient's face.

As a result of the heating and cooling procedure, all heat-treated lenses show some surface defacement that affects optical quality. This warpage can be seen by tilting the lens slightly while holding it out about 6 inches. (Unfortunately, heat treating is still commonly used in some foreign countries. In fact, most do not have an impact-resistance law, a problem since many Americans purchase eyewear while traveling abroad.)

Weight can be a problem where heat-treated lenses are involved. To pass the drop-ball test as outlined in the FDA ruling, optical manufacturers have learned that the lens must have a 2.2mm minimum thickness, except in cases of high plus, where the thick center allows for a slight deviation. Chemically tempered lenses always meet the FDA standards in a thinner form.

Manufacturers in the United States use chemical tempering for plano lenses in sunglass designs; unfortunately, however, since the FDA finds heat treating an acceptable procedure, many foreign manufacturers export sunglasses with lenses made "impact resistant" by this method. These sunfashions are sold to drugstores as over-the-counter products.

Note: There is a problem when photochromics are heat tempered. Heat hardening causes these light-to-dark lenses to lighten slower. It also reduces light transmission indoors. This can be significant enough to be noticed by the wearer.

Occupational Protective Lenses

By definition, an impact-resistant occupational lens is one designed for industrial use. The original standard was as follows: a lens having 3.0mm minimum thickness with the exception of strong plus powers for which 2.5mm minimum thickness was considered adequate. In the test for strength, a $1^1/8$ inch steel ball is dropped freely from a height of 50 inches to the horizontal surface of the lens. Manufacturers have discontinued 3.0mm thickness for almost all plastic lenses because the added thickness is not needed to comply with the testing standards. Research also shows it to be unnecessary for chemically tempered lenses. *Occupational thickness* is a term primarily used when referring to extra-thick, heat-treated glass lenses.

The same heat-treating procedure is used as that involving thinner lenses. After the lens is edged to the desired size and shape, it is brought close to the melting point and then cooled rapidly so that tension is set up between the inner and outer molecular layers of glass. The additional lens thickness usually insures against spontaneous breakage, but the added weight makes it difficult to adjust the glasses comfortably and/or maintain a proper fit.

Unfortunately, a few industries still supply these lenses to their employees, particularly in plano form. Workers often object to the unsightly appearance as well as the discomfort, so manufacturers try to solve some of the problems by limiting the patient's selection to a maximum eyesize of 48 or 50mm. However, their purpose may be defeated, because the small size subtracts from the protective value of the eyewear. In addition, as with all heat-treated lenses, there is surface defacement as a result of curvature distortion. Inexpensive industrial glasses may exhibit this excessively, because tight quality control is not always exercised in their manufacture.

Sometimes patients, particularly women, request industrial lenses be reshaped into a "better-looking" frame. Heat-treated lenses cannot be re-edged without danger of crumbling (2.2mm heat-treated lenses should never be reworked because of the increased possibility of spontaneous breakage). The best answer to this problem is the use of either chemically tempered glass lenses or plastic lenses mounted into attractive frames. More industries are recognizing this logic and are issuing comfortable, well-fitting eyefashions to their employees. Hopefully, all in the near future will recognize that the small additional cost is well worth the advantages.

Note: At one time, 2.0mm to 2.2mm minimum thickness, heat-treated lenses were referred to as *junior case-hardened* or *dress-hardened lenses*; the industrial thickness lenses were called *senior case-hardened* or simply *case-hardened lenses.* Chemical tempering has rendered these terms obsolete.

Fresnel Lenses

The Fresnel lens is actually a plastic membrane, approximately 1mm thick, designed to be attached to an existing conventional plastic or glass lens. It is available in prismatic corrections, plus, and minus powers (see full discussion Chapter 11, "Lenses That Serve Special Needs"). Flexible when held in the hands (it is delivered in a special cardboard holder), the Fresnel membrane is not suitable for wear without the support of another lens. The press-on membrane is placed on the concave surface with water, which provides enough suction to hold it in place. When the Fresnel membrane is attached to a glass lens, the glass does not have to be made impact resistant. If breakage occurs, the Fresnel membrane "holds" the broken pieces. This characteristic simplifies their use for patients undergoing vision therapy. Fresnel lenses are used primarily as loaners intended for short-term wear. Often a number of prescription changes are needed within a short period, and the Fresnel lens can be quickly attached to a non−impact-resistant lens.

Laminated Lenses

Laminated lenses may feature two relatively thin glass lenses bonded together by a cement-type material or two lenses—one glass, the other plastic. The glass does not have to be made impact resistant by heat treating or chemical tempering. If breakage occurs, all or most of the fragments are held intact by the bonding material.

Before the availability of chemical tempering, laminated lenses were used because they offered several advantages over heat-treated lenses. Since they are not subjected to the heating and cooling procedures, the ophthalmic curves remain true. In addition, spontaneous breakage is not a problem, so safety was a consideration in prescribing.

They were also used to obtain uniform color when a deeply tinted, high-power correction was needed. Before the widespread use of colored plastic lenses and glass coatings, most tinted lenses were the result of adding the proper oxide to the ingredients of clear glass. After the tinted blank was readied, the lens was ground to the desired prescription. In minus corrections this produced a lighter center; for a plus prescription the center was darker than the edges; high cylindrical powers resulted in color bands. These color differences became more obvious as the power and/or the size of the lenses increased. To counteract this problem, practitioners prescribed laminated lenses having a plano tinted lens bonded to a clear lens with the proper prescription. (Superior methods of obtaining uniformity for tinted lenses are described in Chapter 9, "Prescribing Absorptive Lenses.")

The older-design laminated lenses have been phased out in the United States. They had a tendency to split apart, and with some high prescriptions, particularly those of minus power, the manufacturing process was too complicated to be feasible. Smaller eyesizes were necessary for comfort (because of the added thickness) and did not always offer adequate protection against the harmful rays of the sun.

Among the greatest improvements in lens design are the newer laminated lenses which can be prescribed without fear of "splitting." By the nature of their construction, all such lenses meet the criteria set by the FDA ruling. Those of ophthalmic quality utilize either plastic or glass lenses, between which a polarizing material is sandwiched. The glass form does not need tempering because broken particles tend to be held intact by the filter.

CONCLUSION

Although chemically tempered lenses have proved to be as impact resistant as those of hard-resin plastic, breakage could result in bits of broken glass becoming imbedded in the eye and surrounding facial tissue. This could result in serious injury. It is always best that plastic lenses be recommended, especially polycarbonates if at all possible. While all patients can benefit from polycarbonate lens designs, they are absolutely critical for the following:

1.   **Monocular patients.** Patients having good vision in only one eye must be prescribed polycarbonate lenses. Since ocular trauma can readily result in blindness, all precautions must be taken, as the likelihood of accidental injury is never predictable.

2.   **Children who wear glasses all or most waking hours.** By nature children are extremely active and often unaware of potential danger that might result in ocular injury. Polycarbonate lenses offer the utmost in safety, comfort, and cosmetic appearance.

3.   **Patients involved in hazardous occupations.** Large industries recognizing the hazardous aspects of various plant operations require impact-resistant lenses. Without exception, insurance coverage for employees hinges on the wearing of specific types of eyewear whenever and wherever it is deemed necessary. However, there are patients, usually self-employed, who do not recognize or acknowledge the possibility of on-the-job ocular injury. It is important, therefore, that the practitioner explore all phases of a patient's occupational and avocational needs so that polycarbonate lenses can be prescribed if a hazard exists.

4.   **Any patient concerned about possible eye complications.** It is not unusual for a practitioner to counsel patients overly concerned about the likelihood of ocular injury. In these cases, prescribing polycarbonate lenses is an assurance that the best protection has been provided.

Although the following research project was conducted decades ago, it is relevant today. The results were published in the June 1968 issue of the *American Journal of Optometry* and in the *Archives of the American Academy of Optometry* and presented a compelling reason for recommending plastic lenses. Titled "Delayed Flaking from Scratches in Glass" and authored by physicist Barry A. J. Clark, the phenomenon presented was that a glass lens does not have to break to be hazardous—scratching alone can present a problem. By the use of microscopic photographs, the delayed-action ejection of small sharp-edged fragments from scratches in glass was studied. It was noted that these fragments are ejected with sufficient velocity to travel to the eyes of spectacle wearers. Although the glass fragments from a scratch on the ocular surface were expelled with velocities much smaller than necessary for penetration into the eyeball, the fragments could lodge between the eyelid and the conjunctiva. Eye movements and blinking would therefore result in abrasion and consequent risk of infection. In addition, the fragments are difficult to remove because of their small size. If the lens was clear (not tinted), transparency hampered the removal process.

Under the same testing conditions, scratches on a CR 39 plastic lens did not result in delayed-action ejection of fragments.

In conclusion the author stated, "It should be clearly understood that the hazard present is of a relatively minor nature when compared with the type and frequency of eye hazards found and is therefore not to be regarded as justification for the nonuse of glass safety spectacles." Nevertheless, the implications are obvious. When the practitioner prescribes an impact-resistant lens, it is the plastic designs that prove the most effective.

Chapter 11

LENSES THAT SERVE SPECIAL NEEDS

INTRODUCTION

There are lens designs that, although limited in use, often serve an important role in the fabrication of eyewear. In some instances they are superior to conventional lenses as constant research results in better cosmetic and/or optical performance.

FRESNEL MEMBRANE PRESS-ON LENSES

The Fresnel press-on membrane is a thin plastic sheet of about 1mm designed to be placed on the ocular surface of an existing glass or plastic lens. It is available in prism corrections, plus and minus full lenses, and a precut plus power straight-top 25mm bifocal-style. Application is quick and simple; water is the only substance needed to hold the membrane in place. (If applied to a glass lens, the lens does not have to be tempered in any way to meet FDA impact-resistance standards. If breakage occurs, the Fresnel membrane will keep the pieces intact.)

Originally distributed by Optical Science Group, Inc., then by Mentor, Fresnel lenses are available through the local laboratory. The membrane is supplied in a squared cardboard carrier. It can be shaped with sharp, high-quality scissors, a razor blade, or by means of specially designed cutting equipment so that it can conform to an existing lens.

Fresnel lenses are rarely worn as a permanent correction because they exhibit several problems. Visual acuity is usually reduced one line by Fresnel optics and all result in a cosmetic loss. Yet, they can serve important roles, as is explained under each type of correction. Since increment steps have varied in the past, it is best to query the laboratory as to availability of powers not given here.

Fresnel Press-on Prisms

The optical principle of the prism Fresnel corrections involves the use of a series of small prisms of equal power whose bases are arranged parallel to each other. The result is a series of parallel lines noticed by both wearer and observer. Fresnel prism powers range from $1/2^\Delta$ to 30^Δ diopters. Unusual prism prescriptions formerly difficult or impossible to fabricate are now easily available by use of the Fresnel press-on membrane. Examples include prism power in bifocal segments and sectional application of prism (i.e., prism in a portion of the lens compensating for a palsied extraocular muscle). Large amounts of prism, such as 15 diopters or greater, can be tolerated since the total eyewear weight is as though no significant prismatic correction was worn. However, as with all Fresnel optics, there is a loss of visual acuity, and cosmesis is adversely affected. The lenses are also difficult to keep clean. The manufacturer recommends rinsing the lens under warm running water and if there is dirt in the multiple grooves, using a soft brush (a baby's toothbrush works well) for removal. The lens should then be blot-dried with a soft, lint-free cloth.

Practically speaking, these lenses are used primarily as temporary corrections for patients undergoing vision therapy. Practitioners specializing in this field find them invaluable in evaluating quickly the amount of prism best serving the patient's needs. Changing the correction is a relatively low-cost procedure, and it takes only minutes to shape the membrane to an existing lens.

Note: The use of Fresnel sectorial prisms in field enhancement for patients who have lost part of their visual field (e.g., strokes, brain tumor, trauma) by projecting the image to the useable portion of the retina has rarely proved successful. The patient tends to become confused trying to orient to a "different" way of seeing. There is also a learning process that may be difficult, even impossible, for a patient who has suffered a physical disability.

Fresnel Membrane Press-on Full Plus Lenses

Full plus Fresnel lenses are easily available in powers +0.50D through +20.00D. The design involves a series of concentric circles. The lower plus powers are used primarily as aids in vision training, but the reduction of visual acuity limits their practicality. At one time the higher powers were used extensively as an interim lens for aphakic patients whose final correction had not been determined. However, since almost all cataract surgery in the United States now involves intraocular lens implants, the higher powers are rarely necessary, except perhaps as a temporary lens if a high plus correction is being fabricated by the laboratory (e.g., lost eyewear).

Fresnel Precut Straight-top 25mm Plus Segments

These add powers ranging from +1.00D to +6.00D and can help evaluate the patient's need for a specific near correction, particularly when a higher power is involved. Some texts recommend the lens as an inexpensive low vision aid, but the resultant drop in visual acuity seriously hinders their value. It is best always to fit conventional lenses for high add prescriptions.

Fresnel Minus Lenses

Minus Fresnel lenses range in power from −1.00D to −14.00D and exhibit a concentric ring pattern. They are sometimes used in vision-training procedures. However, they tend to be more practical as "loaners" to the myope who cannot function without a correction during the time it takes to fabricate conventional eyewear or to receive replacement contact lenses.

Note: For patients who cannot function without a visual correction, the eyecare practitioner should strongly advise the "spare pair." Minus- and plus-power Fresnel lenses are poor substitutes for a prescription that provides clear vision.

HIGH-ADD BIFOCALS FOR LOW-VISION PATIENTS

Patients whose best corrected visual acuity is less than 20/50 may require bifocal adds higher than the +4.00D usually available from the local laboratory. Any conventional fused or one-piece bifocal can be factory-ordered with a higher add. Additions for fused bifocals are usually limited to +4.50D, perhaps, +5.00D because of the increased countersink curve (and the added weight of the higher index glass). Adds as high as +20.00D are available on one-piece bifocals. (Vision-Ease, Inc. is the manufacturer most likely to supply any special-order high add on a glass bifocal.)

Almost any power plus single-vision lens (often used for reading only) is easily available in plastic (much preferable over glass when weight is a serious problem). American Optical makes available plastic microscopic lenses in powers +4.00D to +12.00D in convenient half-eye mountings.

There are special magnifying lenses exclusively designed for the low-vision patient. The best known manufacturer, Designs for Vision, Inc., offers numerous bifocal and trifocal designs. The company should be queried frequently for updates. There are constant improvements upon existing designs as well as the introduction of newer versions to aid the low-vision patient. Prism can even be incorporated if necessary.

It is possible to order cemented add segments placed on single-vision lenses. They are usually fixed on the inside surface but can be ordered on the outside curvature. The segments can be either glass or plastic, but fusion of glass to plastic is not recommended. The newer cements used on the plastic segments do not discolor and dry up with age as they did in the past.

There are a number of advantages in prescribing cemented segments. The most important is versatility. The segment can be ordered in any size and design (round top, flat top, or straight across) with any amount of prism in cases where fusion is a problem. However, most practitioners prefer using the cemented Franklin-style lenses from Designs for Vision, Inc., because local laboratories often are not familiar with the procedures necessary to produce a quality cement-segment bifocal.

HIGH-INDEX LENSES

High-index lenses (higher than crown, 1.523, and CR 39, 1.49) dramatically improve cosmetic appearance, particularly in minus corrections. They have captured great interest in the past few years. Almost every lens manufacturer makes available several high-index, plastic designs.

The original high-index lenses, usually identified as Thinlite or Flintlite, were fashioned of flint glass. Flint has an index of 1.7, so the lenses were thinner than those of standard crown and were recommended for high minus corrections. However, they exhibited several problems. Since flint is relatively heavy, the eyewear tended to be very uncomfortable. In addition, the extreme chromatic aberration and resultant color distortion often annoyed the wearer. Flint lenses were brittle, tending to break more readily than crown. In fact, the FDA ruling regarding impact-resistant lenses made it almost impossible to prescribe them. They could not be made impact resistant, so practitioners fearful of lawsuits hesitated about asking the patient to sign a waiver.

Then a high-index 1.7 glass lens eliminating many of the problems of Flintlite was introduced. Designed primarily for high minus prescriptions, the weight was about that of crown and actually less when the power reached greater than −8.00D. The lens could be made impact resistant by the chemical-tempering method. However, glass can feel heavy on the face, and today high-index plastic lenses are used almost exclusively. Available in index 1.6, 1.7, and 1.8, they are comfortable as well as cosmetically superior to lower-index lenses. In fact, they will soon be so popular they may not belong in a category of lenses for special use. (Aspheric lenses for high powers are discussed later in this chapter.)

X-RAY GLASS LENS

Vision-Ease makes available a high-index 1.8, single-vision, clear lens manufactured of flint glass for use around radiology equipment. Since x-ray radiation can cause serious eye damage, this lens fills a necessary occupational use. It cannot be made impact resistant by chemical treating or heat tempering. However, ordering Corlon polyurethane applied to the back surface can make the lens impact resistant. Specifics can be obtained by querying Vision-Ease, Inc. (If Corlon polyurethane is not ordered, the patient must sign a waiver before this x-ray lens can be prescribed.)

LENSES FOR THE HIGH-PLUS PATIENT

Determining the most suitable lens design for the high-plus patient is a critical consideration. Since the correction is high plus in power, weight is an important factor. So is the optics of the lenses. When the patient looks away from the optical centers, the prismatic effect can result in asthenopia. Cosmesis is always a problem. Facial features viewed through the correction appear considerably magnified and, therefore, distorted.

Fortunately, with the increase of the surgical intraocular lens implant for the cataract patient and the drastic improvement in contact lenses, high-plus spectacle lenses are rarely prescribed. Still for the high-plus patient who wears contacts, a spectacle correction as "back-up" is critical. On days when contacts cannot be worn (the flu, a cold, etc.) vision is so poor the patient can barely function.

Plastic lenses should always be prescribed (to solve the weight problem), and there are important advances in their design. The wide-angle designs, which essentially duplicate the optics of a lenticular style are best (lenticular lenses are discussed later in this chapter). These are called aspherics, and they dramatically improve cosmesis. The lenses look like a conventional design.

ASPHERIC LENSES

There is sometimes confusion as to exactly what are aspheric lenses and how they benefit the patient. Yet probably in no other area has the patient needing a higher power prescription been helped more. The most understood definition of an aspheric lens is one in which the aspheric surface is not a spherical surface. For a plus lens, the front surface of the lens gradually flattens; it is ground steeper for a minus lens. Each manufacturer determines the actual curves for a specific power and promotes the lenses as "the best." However, all have similar optics.

The original aspherics were called Welsh 4-Drop aspherics (designed by R.C. Welsh) because there is approximately 4 diopters less power in the periphery, allowing certain areas of the face to appear more normal. The lenses also give the patient a wider distant field of view. While there may be a drop in visual acuity unless the head is turned, it is less than that resulting from the distortion of a full power high plus lens. In actuality, there is a certain amount of compensation because of the change in vertex distance. Plus powers increase in effectivity when positioned farther away from the pupil, so the periphery has more power than that indicated by the lensometer.

Welsh 4-Drop aspherics were available in a single-vision and two bifocal styles. The straight-top D design had a segment size 22mm × 11mm. This shorter vertical measurement was designed to allow the patient to see beneath the segment for better orientation when walking, climbing stairs, etc. The other bifocal was the round-top 22mm that had its widest area 11mm below the segment line. The latter was not practical because it was difficult to hold the head in a relatively normal position for lengthy reading.

Later a 3-Drop aspheric lens similar in basic construction to the Welsh 4-Drop was released. The power difference from center to edge was about 3 diopters. The newer straight-top D segment was the conventional 22mm × 14mm.

Note: Lenses that feature a round lenticular field are obsolete (Figures 11.1 and 11.2). So is the oval, which featured a useable oval-shaped 45 × 40mm field (Figure 11.3). There are patients who still wear these lenses, and the lenses have to be changed to a more modern design that minimizes the "bulls-eye" effect. The former are illustrated here for recognition purposes.

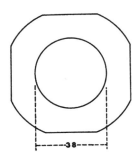

FIGURE 11.1   *Lenticular lens—38mm prescription area (obsolete)*

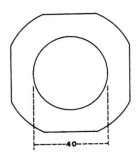

FIGURE 11.2   *Lenticular lens—40mm prescription area (obsolete)*

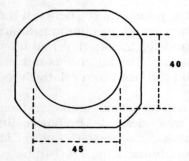

FIGURE 11.3   *45mm × 40mm oval lenticular field (obsolete)*

AVAILABILITY OF ASPHERIC LENSES

Aspheric lenses in glass and plastic are easily available in spherical powers +6.00D to −15.00D (if another power is desired, the local laboratory can be queried).

A newer, high-index plastic, index 1.66, is especially attractive and absorbs ultraviolet (UV) rays to 390nm. It is computer engineered to reduce/eliminate peripheral distortion. The result is a better-looking lens that makes the eye area appear more natural in size. This plastic lens is coated for scratch resistance. Even though it is amazingly thin, the lens will pass the FDA requirement for impact resistance. Query the local laboratory for availability of powers.

Recent advertisements identify a Backside Aspheric (also called *Atoric*) in which the asphericity is applied to the cylindrical surface (back of the lens). Actually an aspheric surface can be either on the spherical or cylindrical side; both result in a more pleasing cosmetic lens, even though usually the aspheric surface is on the front.

Multifocals are also available in aspheric designs. An aspheric bifocal available from Optima is identified as a D-28. The upper division line is very slightly curved (other D-style bifocals have a straight line dividing distance from near). Add power ranges to +3.00D in +.25D steps.

There are also available aspheric progressive addition lenses, a welcomed cosmetic addition to the multifocal field for presbyopic patients needing a high-power prescription. The Hyperview progressive plastic lens has an index of 1.66 and can be tinted to almost any desired shade. It is available in distance powers

−15.00D to +6.00D The full adds range from +.75D to +3.50D. The recommended segment height from the fitting cross to the bottom of the lens is a minimum of 23mm.

The Premier progressive lens is a soft aspheric design, meaning that the peripheral distortion (noted in all progressive addition lenses) is spread out. It is easier for the patient to learn to wear because the rocking motion noted on movement is reduced. The trade-off is less useable true power in the intermediate and near areas.

There undoubtedly will be other bifocal and progressive addition aspheric lenses available soon. The eyecare practitioner can understand the optics by studying the literature that always accompanies each new release.

Whenever possible, it is best to limit the eyesize to about 50mm in an aspheric prescription. The result is less peripheral distortion and a vastly improved cosmetic appearance.

BLENDED MYODISC (YOUNGER OPTICS)

A CR 39 hard-resin, high minus power lens identified as Blended Myodisc is available from Younger Optics. Designed for cosmetic purposes, the edge thickness is reduced by about 40% (over a conventional minus prescription). The design is similar to the 4-Drop aspheric lens for plus prescriptions, basically a lenticular without the lenticular ledges. This means that the peripheral areas are not ground to full power, but this should not be a problem, especially if the lens is ordered for a "small-ish" frame. Blended Myodisc lenses are available in powers ranging from −5.00D sphere to −30.00D sphere. The spherical component is combined with cylinder power up to −2.00D only, but this range may be expanded. The lens is made with special UV absorbers that give specific colors identified as PLS 400, PLS 530, PLS 540, and PLS 550 (see Chapter 9, "Prescribing Absorptive Lenses" for specifics). The Blended Myodisc is a welcomed addition for those desiring an especially attractive high minus lens.

Note: The old Myodisc with a "scooped-out" field and peripheral plano surfaces giving a "bulls-eye" effect should never be prescribed. Patients still wearing this lens can be switched to the Blended Myodisc for better optics and a highly superior cosmetic effect.

Chapter 12

BASE CURVE CONSIDERATIONS

INTRODUCTION

Until recent years, perhaps the most confusing and controversial subject in lens design prescribing was the specification of base curves (curves on front/back of lenses). Most practitioners rarely designated a base curve on a lens prescription, understanding that the designer's academic background and extensive research in the field of ophthalmic optics resulted in lenses having optimum optical performance. In fact, most laboratories will not deviate from the base curves suggested by the manufacturers, especially when oversize, plastic, or photochromic lenses are involved. Sometimes it is a certainty that the ordered curves would adversely affect cosmetic value. In other instances grinding certain curvatures on some lens designs is a procedure too complicated to be feasible. Yet there were academicians who insisted that base curves should be specified. However, lens optics has become so sophisticated that computers now determine curves and that recognition has lessened demand.

In light of what is currently feasible, this chapter will discuss options open to the practitioner as well as give a historical perspective regarding base curves.

BASE CURVES OF SINGLE-VISION LENSES

If a single-vision lens is spherical in correction, the base curve is that curvature common to a series (see Chapter 1, "Characteristics of Lenses"). This definition has remained constant for decades, but within the past decade, defining the base curve for a cylindrical lens has been changing. Manufacturers phased out plus-cylinder, single-vision lenses and discarded the definition that the base curve is the weakest curve on the cylinder surface. Almost without exception, the preferred definition for a minus-cylinder design is that the base curve is the spherical (outside) curvature of the lens.

Every major glass lens manufacturer distributes single-vision and conventional multifocal lenses having specific base curves that correct for certain lens aberrations. Local laboratories stock at least one brand in minus-cylinder corrections and can supply specifics when queried.

Optical experts prefer minus-cylinder lenses because a spherical front surface means that meridional magnification is kept at a minimum. Cosmetic appearance is also more pleasing because curvature changes are on the back surface and therefore less noticeable.

The beginning presbyope who has worn a single-vision inside-surface cylinder design makes the transition from single-vision to multifocal lenses with relative ease. All contemporary multifocals manufactured in the United States (glass and plastic) are made in minus-cylinder form.

HISTORICAL REFERENCE—TRADE NAMES FOR GLASS LENSES HAVING SPECIFIC BASE CURVE CONSTRUCTION

The following identification is given primarily for historical purposes and because reference in texts may still be made to a few of these trade names. Manufacturers may use the term *corrected curve* when referring to quality glass lenses. It has largely been dropped in reference to plastic lenses because it is assumed that all are designed for optimum performance or cosmetic value.

Orthogon Lenses

The Orthogon series of corrected-curve lenses was introduced by Bausch & Lomb, Inc., in 1928. The lenses were ground on any one of 15 base curves, depending on the prescription. All the original designs featured a toric front surface and corrected for radial astigmatism but not for curvature of field.

Tillyer Lenses

The original Tillyer lenses were introduced in 1926 by American Optical Corp. These lenses were ground in plus-cylinder form with the exception of a few minus powers that had a back cylinder design. They featured a partial correction of both marginal astigmatism and curvature of field. The Tillyer name may be retained to designate quality lens designs.

Tillyer Masterpiece

In 1964 the Tillyer Masterpiece lens series was introduced. These lenses, ground in minus-cylinder form, kept meridional magnification at a minimum.

Kurova Lenses

This correct curve series was created by Continental Optical Co. Ground in plus toric form, they were designed to keep marginal astigmatism at a minimum. Eventually, the term *Kurova* was designated as a quality lens (rather than a plus-cylinder form).

Shursite Lenses

These lenses were made available in 1966 by Shuron/Continental. They were ground in minus-cylinder form and designed to keep meridional magnification at a minimum.

Normalsite Lenses

Normalsite lenses, distributed by Titmus Optical Co., were originally manufactured in plus-cylinder form and later replaced by a minus-cylinder construction.

Uniform Lenses

These lenses were created by Univis, Inc. and later distributed under the trade name Best-Form. They were one of the first minus-cylinder designs with meridional magnification kept at a minimum. They were discontinued in 1971.

BASE CURVE OF MULTIFOCALS

The base curve of a multifocal is identified as the spherical distance curvature on the same side as the segment. For all contemporary designs this is the convex (outside) surface of the lens. Specific curvatures can be ascertained by charts available from the various manufacturers. If conventional glass multifocals are prescribed and a different curvature is requested, the base curve can often be altered. The process is more difficult with plastic lenses and few local laboratories will deviate from the manufacturer's designations.

POSSIBLE DEVIATIONS FROM SUGGESTED BASED CURVES

All quality laboratories have trained technicians who can determine what curves will give the best optical and cosmetic effect for a given prescription. As has been previously noted, it is becoming increasingly difficult for the practitioner to deviate from these recommendations, yet there are times when attempts to do so may be necessary.

If the lens powers for a given prescription are drastically different for each eye, specifying that the outside curves be approximately the same is a critical cosmetic factor.

A practitioner may feel that when a patient has adjusted to specific base curves, curvatures should be duplicated. However, with today's lens and frame designs, this theory is difficult to follow. If glasses have been worn, particularly those having a high correction, when the curves are changed, the patient should be advised of the possibility of an adjustment period (usually a few weeks). Some patients are sensitive to changes in base curve if they alternate between more than one pair. For example, a patient may wear an outdoor correction having plastic lenses and an indoor prescription utilizing glass lenses. The curvatures may not be the same. Whenever possible, it is best to recommend lenses with similar base curves.

A problem can arise from the use of minus cylinder, single-vision glass lenses. Since they are ground with relatively flat curves, the patient with long lashes and/or a flat bridge may find that the lashes touch the lenses. A deeper lens can be ordered (i.e., +8.00 or +9.00D outside curvature), but this often means sacrificing cosmetic appearance. Fortunately, many attractive contemporary frames are available with an adjustable pad bridge construction so they can be positioned properly; alternatively, the patient may prefer to slide the eyewear slightly down the nose.

It is wise to clock lenses with the Geneva Lens Gauge when the eyewear is received from the laboratory and to record the base curves. Sometimes a change in curvature is a continuing annoyance to the patient; such knowledge is helpful when pin-pointing possible sources of problems. In very rare cases it may be necessary to change back to lenses duplicating the original base curves.

BALANCE LENS

It may be good to mention here the ordering of a balance lens for the patient whose vision cannot be improved in one eye. If "balance lens" is written on the prescription form, the laboratory may use any available discarded lens. For cosmetic effect, the balance lens should be ordered close to the prescription for the other eye and in the same lens design. Eyewear is not attractive if, for instance, the patient wears a flat-top, D-style bifocal before the right eye and a single-vision lens in front of the left.

FRONT SURFACE CURVATURE AND LENS MAGNIFICATION

There may be instances when the practitioner wishes to know the magnification created by a lens. Magnification or image size depends upon the following four factors. The first of these factors is unalterable; the other three can be controlled.

1. Power of the lens
2. Front surface curvature (this variable contributes the most to magnification effects)
3. Lens thickness
4. Vertex distance

Magnification is computed using the following formulas:

$$M_p = \frac{1}{1 - hD_v}$$

M_p = magnification as a result of the power

$$M_s = \frac{1}{1 - D_1(t/n)}$$

H = vertex distance
D_v = vertex power
M_s = magnification as a result of the shape of the lens
D_1 = power of the front curve
t = thickness in meters of the lens
n = index of the lens

$$M_{total} = M_p \times M_s$$
$$M_{total} = \text{total magnification}$$
$$\% = (M_{total} - 1) \times 100\%$$

The answer is stated in percentage of magnification.

PROBLEM:

A 45mm round lens of +2.00D power is worn 16mm anterior to the cornea. This lens has a +8.00D front surface, a −6.00D ocular surface, and is 2.5mm thick (center position). What is the magnification produced by the lens?

PROCEDURE:

1.   Determine the magnification as a result of the power.

$$M_p = \frac{1}{1 - hD_v}$$

$$= \frac{1}{1 - (0.016)(+2)}$$

$$= 1.03$$

2. Determine the magnification due to the shape.

$$M_s = \frac{1}{1 - (t/n)\ D_1}$$

$$= \frac{1}{1 - (0.0025\ /\ 1.523)(8)}$$

$$= 1.01$$

3. Determine total magnification.

$$M_{total} = M_p \times M_s$$

$$= 1.03 \times 1.01$$

$$= 1.04$$

4.

$$\% = (M_{total} - 1) \times 100\%$$

$$= (1.04 - 1) \times 100\%$$

$$= 4\%$$

SOLUTION:

Magnification = 4%.

PROBLEM:

What is the magnification of a +3.00D spherical lens constructed with a +6.00D front surface and center thickness of 2mm, and worn with the back vertex 17mm from the entrance pupil of the eye?

PROCEDURE:

1. Determine the magnification as a result of the power.

$$M_p = \frac{1}{1 - (0.017)(+3)}$$

$$= 1.05$$

2.   Determine the magnification due to the shape.

$$M_s = \frac{1}{1-(0.002\,/\,1.523)(6)}$$

$$= \frac{1}{0.992}$$

$$= 1.008$$

3.   Determine total magnification.

$$M_{total} = 1.05 \times 1.008$$

$$= 1.058$$

4.

$$\% = (M_{total} - 1) \times 100\%$$
$$= (1.058 - 1) \times 100\%$$
$$= 5.8\%$$

SOLUTION:

Magnification = 5.8%

A practitioner who wishes to equalize the magnification of two lenses can do so by changing the front curvature of one lens. Two problems follow as examples of how this is accomplished.

PROBLEM:

A patient wears a pair of spectacles 15mm anterior to the corneal vertex The left lens is a +2.00D sphere with 2.5mm center thickness. The right lens is +3.00D with 3.0mm center thickness and has a front curvature of +6.00D. The index of the lenses is 1.52. Determine the front curvature of the left lens if both lenses are to have equal magnification.

SOLUTION:

1. Determine magnification of the right lens.

$$M_p = \frac{1}{1 - hD_v}$$

$$= \frac{1}{1 - (0.015)(3)} = \frac{1}{0.955}$$

$$= 1.046$$

$$M_s = \frac{1}{1 - t/n \ (D_1)}$$

$$= \frac{1}{1 - (0.003/1.52)(6)} = \frac{1}{0.988}$$

$$= 1.01$$

$$M_{total} = 1.046 \times 1.01 = 1.056$$

$$\% = (1.056 - 1.00) \times 100\% = 5.6$$

2. Determine magnification as a result of the power of the left lens.

$$M_p = \frac{1}{1 - hD_v}$$

$$= \frac{1}{1 - (0.015)(2)} = \frac{1}{0.97}$$

$$= 1.03$$

3. Determine magnification needed from shape factor for the right lens.

$$M_{total} = M_p \times M_s$$

$$M_s = \frac{1.056}{1.03}$$

$$= 1.02$$

4. Solve for front curvature of right lens.

$$M_s = \frac{1}{1 - t/n \ (D_1)}$$

$$1.02 = \frac{1}{1 - (0.0025/1.52)D_1}$$

$$1.02 - 0.00163D_1 = 1$$

$$0.00163D_1 = 0.02$$

$$D_1 = +12.00D$$

SOLUTION:

Front surface of left lens needs to be +12.00D to equalize magnification.

PROBLEM:

A patient requires the following prescription:
              O.D. + 4.00 D.S.
              O.S. + 3.00 D.S.
The center thickness of the right lens is 3.5mm. The front curve is +10.00D. The center thickness of the left lens is 3.5mm. The lens index is 1.52; the vertex distance is 12mm. Calculate the front curvature of the left lens necessary to equalize the magnification.

PROCEDURE:

1. Determine M_{total} for right lens.

$$M_p = \frac{1}{1 - hD_v}$$

$$= \frac{1}{1 - (0.012)(4)} = \frac{1}{0.952}$$

$$= 1.05$$

$$M_s = \frac{1}{1 - t/n \ (D_1)}$$

$$= \frac{1}{1 - (0.0035/1.52)(10)} = \frac{1}{0.977}$$

$$= 1.02$$

$$M_{total} = 1.05 \times 1.02 = 1.07$$

$$\% = (1.07 - 1.00) \times 100\%$$

$$= 7\%$$

2. Determine M_p for left lens.

$$M_p = \frac{1}{1 - hD_v}$$

$$= \frac{1}{1 - (0.012)(3)} = \frac{1}{0.964}$$

$$= 1.03$$

3. Determine M_s for left lens.

$$M_s = \frac{1.07}{1.03}$$

$$= 1.04$$

4.   Determine D_1 for left lens.

$$1.04 = \frac{1}{1 - (0.0035/1.52)D_1}$$

$$1.04 - 0.0024D_1 = 1$$

$$0.0024D_1 = 0.04$$

$$D_1 = +16.66D$$

SOLUTION:

The front curvature of the left lens needs to be +16.62D (the closest 0.12D) to equalize magnification.

Chapter 13

VERTICAL IMBALANCE AT THE READING LEVEL

INTRODUCTION

When a patient looks beneath the distance optical centers of lenses having different powers in the vertical meridians, prismatic imbalance results. If the imbalance is $1^{1}/_{2}$ prism diopters or more, the practitioner needs to be aware of possible symptoms, such as a pulling sensation "when I read," doubling when reading, and/or headaches usually in the frontal area.

Vertical prismatic imbalance is best eliminated by wearing contact lenses. Recent advances in contact lens design makes it possible to fit almost every patient needing single-vision lenses and should be seriously considered. If for some reason, contact lenses are not an option, bicentric grinding (slab off) is the only possible procedure when a single-vision correction is involved. Until 1986, the two optical centers were created in the lens having the highest minus or lowest plus power (to counteract the prism base-down effect). Then Younger Optics introduced a plastic CR 39, slab off, molded with prism base down on the front surface of the blank. It is placed on the most plus (least minus) lens. Both methods result in a slab-off line that extends from the temporal to the nasal extremities of the lens. Its appearance is similar to that of a straight-across bifocal, and its height is determined in the same manner as that of a conventional straight-top bifocal (usually 1mm below the lower lid).

Vertical prismatic imbalance in a bifocal correction can be compensated for by the slab-off procedure either by the conventional method or by Younger Optics' reverse slab off (made in flat-top 25mm and 28mm and now also available from Vision-Ease). Prescribing bifocal segments having optical centers varying in position or using segments having the compensating prism ground into them is also possible, but these two methods have been made obsolete by the efficiency of bicentric grinding (also known as the *slab-off procedure*).

When it is necessary to compensate for vertical prismatic imbalance in a trifocal correction, the conventional slab-off method is the only possible procedure (placed on the highest minus).

BICENTRIC GRINDING IN A SINGLE-VISION PRESCRIPTION

With the advance in contact lens design, it is rare to correct for vertical imbalance in a single-vision prescription. If conventional single-vision lenses are prescribed, usually the patient is instructed to hold reading material in a relatively straightforward position. This enables the patient to look just below the optical centers of the lenses when focusing at the near point.

In cases where the patient's visual tasks do not make this possible, a slab-off correction is prescribed. To determine the amount, it is first necessary to compute the vertical prismatic imbalance at the reading level. It is assumed that the patient reads 8mm below the distance optical centers of the lenses unless otherwise measured.

PROBLEM:

A patient requires the following prescription:

O.D. +4.00D.S.
O.S. +1.00D.S.

A decision is made to prescribe a slab-off lens. How would this correction be ordered from the laboratory?

PROCEDURE:

1. The formula for determining vertical imbalance is the Prentice prism formula.

    $$\text{Vertical imbalance} = F_v \text{ (cm)}$$

    F_v = difference in power between the vertical meridians of the two lenses.

    cm = distance from the optical centers of the lenses to the reading point.

2. Vertical imbalance = $+4.00 - (+1.00) \times 0.8$cm
    $$= 2.4^\Delta$$

3. Slab-off is ordered in $1/2^\Delta$ steps rounded off to the lowest half.

SOLUTION:

Slab-off 2^Δ O.S. at 14mm high (height arbitrarily determined for demonstration).
    Special Note: If the Younger Optics reverse slab-off lenses (available in CR 39 only) are used, the slab-off correction is 2^Δ on the *right* lens.

PROBLEM:

A patient wears the following correction:

O.D. +6.00 −2.00 × 45°
O.S. +2.00 −4.00 × 30°

If bicentric grinding is required, what is ordered from the laboratory? The patient reads 7mm below the distance optical centers.

PROCEDURE:

1. Determine the power in the vertical meridian of each lens.

    O.D. $+6.00 + (1/2)(-2.00) = +5.00$D
    O.S. $+2.00 + (3/4)(-4.00) = -1.00$D

2. Determine the difference in lens power.

$$+5.00 - (-1.00) = 6.00D$$

3. Compute the amount of vertical imbalance.

$$V.I. = F_v(cm)$$
$$= 6 \times 0.7$$
$$= 4.2^\Delta$$

Overcompensation is not desired, so the slab-off correction is rounded to the lowest $1/2$ prism diopter (ordered in $1/2$ prism diopter steps).

SOLUTION:

Slab-off 4^Δ O.S. at 14mm high (height arbitrarily determined for demonstration purposes).
    Note: The Younger Optics reverse slab-off correction is 4^Δ O.D.

PROBLEM:

Given the following prescription:
    O.D. +3.00 −2.00 × 45°
    O.S. plano −4.00 × 90°
If the patient reads 8mm below the distance optical centers, what is the slab-off correction ordered from the laboratory?

PROCEDURE:

1. Determine the power in the vertical meridian of each lens.

$$O.D. +3.00 + (1/2) (-2.00) = +2.00D$$
$$O.S. 0.00 + (0) (-4.00) = 0.00D$$

2. Determine the difference in lens powers.

$$+2.00 - 0.00 = 2.00D$$

3. Compute the amount of vertical imbalance.

$$V.I. = F_v(cm)$$
$$= 2 (0.8)$$
$$= 1.6^\Delta$$

SOLUTION:

Slab-off 1.5$^\Delta$ O.S. (measured height; i.e., 15mm high) or Younger Optics reverse slab-off, 1.5$^\Delta$ O.D.

Note: Practically speaking, this imbalance is too small to give rise to symptoms, so a correction is unnecessary.

PROBLEM:

The following lenses are prescribed

$$\text{O.D. } -1.00 \ -5.00 \times 180°$$
$$\text{O.S. } -2.00 \text{ D.S.}$$

The patient reads 7mm below the optical centers. How is the bicentric grinding ordered?

PROCEDURE:

1. Determine the power in the vertical meridian of each lens.

$$\text{O.D. } -1.00 + (1) \ (-5.00) = -6.00\text{D}$$
$$\text{O.S. } -2.00 \text{ D.S.}$$

2. Determine the difference in lens powers.

$$-6.00 - (-2.00) = -4.00\text{D}$$

3. Compute the vertical imbalance.

$$\text{V.I.} = F_v(\text{cm})$$
$$= 4 \ (.7)$$
$$= 2.8^\Delta$$

SOLUTION:

Slab-off 2.5$^\Delta$ O.D. (at the measured height; i.e., 14mm high) or 2.5$^\Delta$ O.S. for Younger Optics reverse slab-off.

SLAB-OFF IN A BIFOCAL PRESCRIPTION

There are a number of methods used to compensate for vertical imbalance at the reading level in a bifocal correction. The most practical method is the slab-off procedure. From a cosmetic viewpoint it is the most pleasing, because the slab off coincides with the segment dividing line.

Therefore, flat-top segments are best (also called straight-top segments or D segments). The larger the segment the less obvious is the slab-off line (because it coincides with the top of the segment). Practitioners tend to prefer the FT–28mm style because in most cases, it serves well as a general-purpose bifocal.

For ordering bicentric grinding in a bifocal correction, the procedure is the same as that used with a single-vision correction. The add power at near does not affect the amount of vertical imbalance because it is the same for both eyes.

PROBLEM:

A patient wears the following prescription:

O.D. +6.00 −2.00 × 45°
O.S. +3.00 −2.00 × 30°
O.U. Add +2.00D

Flat-top 28mm bifocal style set at 14mm high.
If the patient reads 8mm below the distance optical centers, what would be the bicentric grinding ordered from the laboratory?
(Unless there is a specific reason to measure otherwise, it is assumed patients read 8mm below the distance optical centers, since the slab off does not have to fully correct for vertical imbalance.)

PROCEDURE:

1. Determine the power in the vertical meridian of each lens.

O.D. +6.00 + ($1/2$) (−2.00) = +5.00D
O.S. +3.00 + ($3/4$) (−2.00) = +1.50D

2. Determine the vertical imbalance.

V.I. = (+5.00 − 1.50) (0.8)
= 2.8$^\Delta$

SOLUTION:

Slab off 2.5$^\Delta$ O.S. at 14mm high to coincide with the segment height, or Younger Optics reverse slab off 2.5$^\Delta$ O.D. (Correction is lowered to the closest $1/2^\Delta$.)

SLAB OFF OR BICENTRIC GRINDING IN A TRIFOCAL CORRECTION

The amount of slab off in a trifocal correction is computed and ordered in the same manner as that of a bifocal prescription. Since the intermediate and near adds are equal for each eye, the compensation is for the imbalance caused by the difference in distance power between the two lenses. A flat-top (straight-top) trifocal design should always be used. It is best to order the slab-off line coinciding with the division between the near and intermediate segments, although it can be placed at the separation between the intermediate and distance if desired.

PROBLEM:

A patient needs the following trifocal prescription:

$$\text{O.D. } -5.00 - .50 \times 180°$$
$$\text{O.S. } -2.00 - 1.50 \times 45°$$
$$\text{O.U. Add } +2.50D$$

An ST 7–28mm trifocal lens is prescribed with an overall segment height of 22mm. If the patient reads 12mm below the distance optical centers, what would be the bicentric grinding ordered from the laboratory? (The 12mm is a logical assumption.)

SOLUTION:

1. Determine the power in the vertical meridian of each lens.

$$\text{O.D. } -5.00 + (-0.50) = -5.50D$$
$$\text{O.S. } -2.00 + (^1\!/_2)(-1.00) = -2.50D$$

2. Determine the difference in lens power.

$$-5.50 - (-2.50) = -3.00D$$

3. Compute the amount of vertical imbalance.

$$\text{V.I. } = F_v(\text{cm})$$
$$= 3 \times 1.2$$
$$= 3.6^\Delta$$

ANSWER:

Correction is rounded to the lowest $^1\!/_2$ prism diopter; slab off 3.5^Δ O.D. (highest minus) at 15mm high. Total segment height is 22mm; intermediate segment is 7mm high. Height of near segment is 22mm – 7mm, or 15mm high; slab-off line will coincide with division between near and intermediate segments. (Not a reverse slab off.)

Special Notes Regarding Bicentric Grinding (Slab-off Corrections)

1. **In past years, local laboratories designed and made most slab-off corrections.** The result was high breakage and a slab-off that was "wavy." Vision-Ease now stocks conventional glass bicentric semifinished blanks in all straight-top segment styles. The slab-off line is always straight; there is faster service and a more reliable delivery date. Available powers are $1^1/_2$ prism diopters to 6 prism diopters. Vision-Ease will also make any bicentric lens (power, tint, etc.) on special order and calculate the amount of prism if the practitioner desires that service. This includes Executive-type corrections, which many local laboratories hesitated to supply because of difficulty in processing.

2. **The Younger slab-off series made in CR 39 only is available in $1^1/_2$ prism diopter to 6 prism diopter corrections in single-vision and two bifocal styles,** ST25mm and ST28mm (flat-top). There are also special UV-absorbing lenses available. This excellent form of bicentric correction must involve an explanation to the patient wearing a conventional slab-off lens; otherwise it is easy to assume that the correction was placed on the wrong lens.

3. **Probably the best solution for patients needing two drastically different corrections in each eye is to recommend contact lenses,** the use of which eliminates vertical imbalance. If a near correction is needed, the lenses then would be of the same power.

Note: The term *double slab off* sometimes seen in texts does not apply to a correction for vertical imbalance. At one time this procedure was used to reduce the lower edge thickness of high-minus lenses, but the resultant slab-off lines on both lenses made the cosmetic value doubtful. High-index plastic lenses now available are the recognized cosmetic solution.

CHECKING THE AMOUNT OF SLAB-OFF ON A LENS

For checking a slab-off prescription, the amount of bicentric grinding is easily determined by using the Geneva lens measure.

1. Place the three pins of the gauge horizontally on the surface with the bicentric grinding. They are positioned just above the slab-off line (Figure 13.1).
2. Note the reading on the gauge.
3. Hold the gauge vertically with the center pin on the slab-off line (Figure 13.2).
4. Note the reading on the gauge.
5. The difference between the two readings is the amount of bicentric grinding.

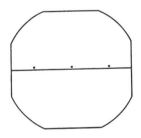

FIGURE 13.1   *Slab-off line*

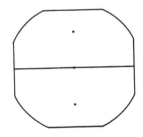

FIGURE 13.2   *Slab-off line*

Example:

With the pins positioned horizontally, the reading is +6.50D. The reading with the gauge held vertically is +10.00D. Therefore, the amount of slab-off is $3^1/2^\Delta$ [+10.00D (−) +6.50D].

DISSIMILAR BIFOCAL SEGMENTS

The use of dissimilar segments with varying optical centers is an obsolete method for correcting vertical imbalance in a bifocal prescription. However, there are still available two possibilities.

One involves the use of R-compensated segments. These designs were originated by Univis, Inc., and are currently available from Vision-Ease (in glass only). The other involves different-size round-top (also known as Ultex), one-piece bifocals. Although these techniques have been made obsolete by slab-off grinding, the lenses are discussed here, not as recommended corrections but because a few geriatric patients having worn R-compensating segments for decades cling to the former method, and the latter is an accepted procedure in some parts of the world.

Vertical imbalance is eliminated or decreased by selecting two proper correcting segments, one of which has a low optical center (base-up prism). To counteract unwanted prism at near, one style is placed before the right eye, the other before the left. The result is not cosmetically pleasing because the appearance of each bifocal differs drastically. It is unusual for more than $1^1/_2$ prism diopters to be corrected by this method. Since patients rarely experience problems until the imbalance exceeds that amount, the use of dissimilar segments is only a partial correction but was thought to be enough to alleviate symptoms (slab off corrects the necessary amount).

R-Compensating Segments

Univis, Inc. created the R series of compensating bifocals. They are now available from Vision-Ease (in glass only). Since each prescription is custom made, the horizontal can be ordered 28mm or 26mm wide. All segments, however, measure 14mm vertically. The series consist of seven segments, each designated by the number that corresponds to optical-center positioning. The range is #4 to #10. The upper and lower limits of each bifocal are straight lines varying in length.

The #4 has an optical center that is 4mm below the upper segment line with the upper division longer than the lower (Figure 13.3).

In the #5 and #6 designs the upper line is also longer than the lower but not as long as the R #4 (Figures 13.4 and 13.5).

Since the #7 is the conventional R bifocal with the optical center halfway between, the top and bottom lines are equal (Figure 13.6).

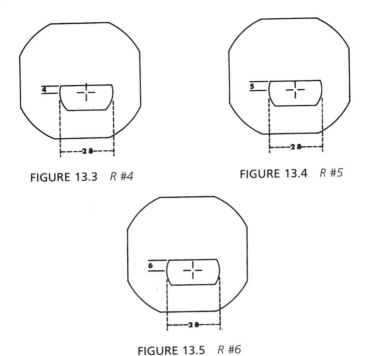

FIGURE 13.3   *R #4*   FIGURE 13.4   *R #5*

FIGURE 13.5   *R #6*

The #8 and #9 designs reverse the pattern with the lower line longer than the upper (Figures 13.7 and 13.8). The lower line reaches its maximum length in the R #10 design (Figure 13.9).

For compensating for vertical imbalance, the segment with the lowest optical center (for its base-down effect) is placed over the lens having the higher plus power.

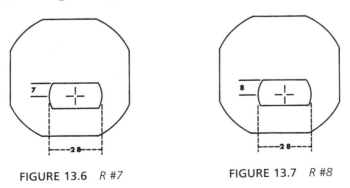

FIGURE 13.6   *R #7*   FIGURE 13.7   *R #8*

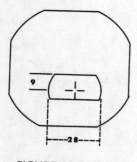

FIGURE 13.8   R #9

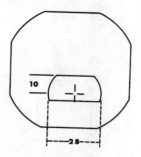

FIGURE 13.9   R #10

PROBLEM:

Given the following prescription:

O.D. $+1.00 - 1.00 \times 45°$
O.S. $-1.00 - 1.00 \times 30°$
O.U. Add $+3.00$D

The patient reads 8mm below the distance optical centers. Which of the lenses in the R-compensated series would correct the vertical imbalance?

PROCEDURE:

1. Determine the power in the meridian of each lens.

    O.D. $+1.00 + (^1/_2) (-1.00) = +0.50$D
    O.S. $-1.00 + (^3/_4) (-1.00) = -1.75$D

2. Determine the vertical imbalance.

    V.I. $= (+.50 - 1.75) (0.8)$
    $= 1.8^\Delta$

3. Compute the separation of the segment optical centers necessary to compensate for the vertical imbalance.

$$x = \frac{V.I.}{Add}$$

$$= \frac{1.8}{3.00}$$

$$= 0.6cm = 6mm$$

SOLUTION:

The following combination will correct the vertical imbalance:

O.D. R-compensating segment #10
O.S. R-compensating segment #4

Note: Again to emphasize, slab off is a better solution for correction of vertical imbalance.

Ultex-Style One-Piece Round-top Bifocals

The other method of compensating for vertical imbalance using dissimilar segments involves prescribing two different sized Ultex-style one-piece, round-top bifocals. This method is not used in the United States. While the conventional Ultex E is no longer available here, it is available in other parts of the world.

There are four lens designs in this series (the term *Ultex* is retained by common usage):

Ultex B—Optical center 11mm down from the dividing line (22mm across)

Ultex E—O.C. 16mm down from the dividing line (32mm across)

Ultex A—O.C. 19mm down from the dividing line (36mm across)

Kingsize Ultex—O.C. 20mm down from the dividing line (40mm across)

PROBLEM:

Given the following prescription:

O.D. −2.00 − 1.00 × 30°
O.S. −0.50 − .050 × 45°
O.U. Add +3.00D

The patient reads 8mm below the distance optical center. Compensate for the vertical imbalance using Ultex-style one-piece round-top segments.

PROCEDURE:

1. Determine the power in the vertical meridian of each lens.

O.D. −2.00 +($3/4$) (−1.00) = −2.75D
O.S. −0.50 + ($1/2$) (−0.50) = −0.75D

2.   Determine the vertical imbalance.

$$V.I. = [-2.75 - (-0.75)] \, (0.8)$$
$$= 1.6^{\Delta}$$

3.   Compensate the separation of the segment optical centers necessary to compensate for the vertical imbalance.

$$x = \frac{V.I.}{Add}$$

$$= \frac{1.6}{3.00}$$

$$= 0.5cm = 5mm \text{ separation}$$

SOLUTION:

The following lenses will correct the vertical imbalance:
O.D. Ultex B (O.C. 11mm down from top of segment)
O.S. Ultex E (O.C. 16mm down from top of segment)
    Note: Problem is given for historical value only. Slab off is always a better solution.

PRISM SEGMENTS

Prism segments should never be used to correct vertical imbalance (counteracting imbalance by prism ground into the segments). This method is highly impractical for several reasons. Prism segments are most unattractive; there is pronounced distortion when the patient looks through the segments; the prism limits the near field of view. The procedure is mentioned here only to acquaint the reader with the disadvantages because it is described in publications involving compensations for vertical imbalance. The following example is given for clarity in understanding how it works and must not be construed as an example of how to prescribe. In fact, it is unlikely that segments with prism base-up/base-down are available in the United States. They are made in Europe but likely by now are discontinued. The last designs in the United States with these possibilities were Panoptik prism segments manufactured by Bausch & Lomb, Inc., who have discontinued production of all prescription ophthalmic lenses.

PROBLEM:

Given the following prescription:

O.D. +4.00 D.S.
O.S. +2.00 D.S.
O.U. Add +2.00D

The patient reads 7mm below the distance optical centers. Compensate for the vertical imbalance at the near point using prism segments.

PROCEDURE:

1.   Determine the amount of vertical imbalance.

$$V.I. = (4.00 - 2.00)(0.7)$$
$$= 1.4^\Delta$$

2.   Therefore compensation is for 1^Δ (rounded off to the lowest $1/2^\Delta$).

SOLUTION:

(For illustration purpose only)
$1/2^\Delta$ BD over O.D.; $1/2^\Delta$ BU over O.S. (divided equally between the two lenses).

Obviously, this problem serves only as an illustration; in any case, the amount of vertical imbalance is too small for a necessary compensation.

Chapter 14

PRESCRIPTION CHANGES INDUCED BY LENS TILT

INTRODUCTION

Modern frames are manufactured or fit so that the lower edges are angled in toward the cheeks. Positioning the glasses thus allows the eyewear to closely follow facial lines. (The term *glasses* continues from common usage although plastic designs are the overwhelming choice for ophthalmic lenses.)

The angle between the vertical plane of the face and the positioning of the glasses, normally between 5° and 10°, is known as the pantoscopic tilt or pantoscopic angle.

Note: Theoretically, a retroscopic angle is one in which the lower edges of the frame are angled away from the vertical plane of the face. However, an actual retroscopic tilt is not used in the fitting of eyewear. The term is used clinically to designate a decrease in the pantoscopic angle.

CHANGE IN EFFECTIVE POWER

When a patient looks away from the optical center of a lens, an aberration known as *oblique* or *marginal astigmatism* is induced. Manufacturers of quality lenses usually correct this aberration for a line of sight passing 30° away from the optical center of the lens. However, as a result of the pantoscopic tilt, the correction for marginal astigmatism is nullified when the patient looks below the optical center.

If the lens power is low, the change in effective power is insignificant. When a higher power is involved, the pantoscopic angle may result in a prescription change critical to the patient.

When a spherical lens is tilted, two changes take place. The result is a new spherical power and the introduction of a cylinder power the axis of which is in the meridian of rotation. Since a pantoscopic angle is a tilt in the horizontal meridian, the resultant axis is 180°.

If a sphero-cylinder lens is tilted pantoscopically, the result is a new spherical power and a different cylinder power.

POWER CHANGES WHEN A PANTOSCOPIC TILT IS INVOLVED

When a lens is tilted pantoscopically, the change in power depends on two factors:

1.   The power of the lens in the vertical meridian.
2.   The angle of the tilt.

As the lens power and/or the angle increases, there is a greater increase in the power change. Two formulas describe the power variation: The first determines change in the spherical correction; the second determines the amount of induced cylinder.

$$F_{\text{new sphere}} = F_{\text{original sphere}} \left(1 + 1/3 \sin^2 \Theta\right)$$

Θ is the angle of tilt from the vertical plane

$$F_{\text{induced cylinder}} = F_{\text{original sphere}} \left(\tan^2 \Theta\right)$$

The induced cylinder has the same sign as the power in the meridian involved. A plus sphere induces a plus cylinder while a minus sphere results in the introduction of a minus cylinder. Since the axis of the induced cylinder is in the meridian of rotation, it is 180°.

PROBLEM:

A +3.00D sphere is tilted pantoscopically 20°. What is the resultant prescription?

PROCEDURE:

1. Determine power of the new sphere.

$$F_{n.s.} = F_{o.s.}(1 + \tfrac{1}{3}\sin^2 \Theta$$
$$= +3.00(1 + \tfrac{1}{3}\sin^2 20)$$
$$= +3.117D$$

2. Determine power of the induced cylinder.

$$F_{i.c.} = F_{o.s.}(\tan^2 \Theta)$$
$$= +3.00(\tan^2 20°)$$
$$= +0.396D$$

3. Combine (1) and (2).

SOLUTION:

$$+3.117D + 0.396D \times 180°$$

PROBLEM:

A $-4.00D$ sphere is angled pantoscopically 15°. Find the new effective power.

PROCEDURE:

1. Determine the power of the new sphere.

$$F_{n.s.} = F_{o.s.}(1 + \tfrac{1}{3}\sin^2 \Theta)$$
$$= -4.00(1 + \tfrac{1}{3}\sin^2 15°)$$
$$= -4.088D$$

2. Determine the power of the induced cylinder.

$$F_{i.c.} = F_{o.s.}(\tan^2 \Theta)$$
$$= -4.00(\tan^2 15°)$$
$$= -0.288D$$

3.   Combine (1) and (2).

SOLUTION:

−4.088D − 0.288D × 180°
The above problems show only a small prescription change. Although there is a large angle of tilt, the lens powers are not high.

PROBLEM:

A +7.00D sphere is angled pantoscopically 15°. Find the new effective power.

PROCEDURE:

1.   Determine the power of the new sphere.

$$F_{n.s.} = F_{o.s.}(1 + \tfrac{1}{3}\sin^2 \Theta)$$
$$= +7.00(1 + \tfrac{1}{3}\sin^2 15°)$$
$$= +7.154D$$

2.   Determine the power of the induced cylinder.

$$F_{i.c.} = F_{o.s.}(\tan^2 \Theta)$$
$$= +7.00(\tan^2 15°)$$
$$= +0.504D$$

3.   Combine (1) and (2).

SOLUTION:

+7.154D + 0.504D × 180°

PROBLEM:

A −6.00D sphere is tilted pantoscopically 20°. What is the new effective power?

PROCEDURE:

1. Determine the power of the new sphere.

$$F_{n.s.} = F_{o.s.}(1 + \tfrac{1}{3}\sin^2 \Theta)$$
$$= -6.00(1 + \tfrac{1}{3}\sin^2 20°)$$
$$= -6.234D$$

2. Determine the power of the induced cylinder.

$$F_{i.c.} = F_{o.s.}(\tan^2 \Theta)$$
$$= -6.00(\tan^2 20°)$$
$$= -0.792D$$

3. Combine (1) and (2).

SOLUTION:

$-6.234D - 0.792D \times 180°$
The above two problems show a prescription change that may be significant to the patient.

PROBLEM:

A lens of $+14.00D$ is tilted pantoscopically $20°$. What is the resultant effective power?

PROCEDURE:

1. Determine the power of the new sphere.

$$F_{n.s.} = F_{o.s.}(1 + \tfrac{1}{3}\sin^2 \Theta)$$
$$= +14.00(1 + \tfrac{1}{3}\sin^2 20°)$$
$$= +14.566D$$

2.   Determine the power of the induced cylinder.

$$F_{i.c.} = F_{o.s.}(\tan^2 \Theta)$$

$$= +14.00(\tan^2 20°)$$

$$= +1.848D$$

3.   Combine (1) and (2).

SOLUTION:

$+14.566D + 1.848D \times 180°$
This problem demonstrates that a high-power lens having a large pantoscopic tilt results in a prescription change that can be disturbing to the patient.

TILTING OF SPHERO-CYLINDER CORRECTIONS

If the original prescription includes a cylinder, only the total power in the vertical meridian is affected by the pantoscopic tilt. The power in the vertical meridian, therefore, is used to calculate the newly induced sphere and cylinder.

To determine the final effective power, the original cylinder is combined with the induced changes, as illustrated in the following examples.

PROBLEM:

A lens of $+5.00 - 1.00 \times 90°$ is tilted pantoscopically 15°. What is the resultant effective power?

PROCEDURE:

Since the cylinder axis is 90°, the total cylinder power is in the 180° meridian. Therefore, the cylinder in this example does not affect the total power in the vertical meridian.

1.   Determine the power of the new sphere.

$$F_{n.s.} = F_{o.s.}(1 + {}^1\!/_3 \sin^2 \Theta)$$

$$= +5.00(1 + {}^1\!/_3 \sin^2 15°)$$

$$= +5.11D$$

2.   Determine the power of the induced cylinder.

$$F_{i.c.} = F_{o.s.}(\tan^2 \Theta)$$

$$= +5.00(\tan^2 15°)$$

$$= +0.36D$$

3.   The induced power is $+5.11 + 0.36 \times 180°$; transposed it is $+5.47 - 0.36 \times 90°$.

4.   Combine with original cylinder.

$$
\begin{array}{r}
+5.47 - 0.36 \times 90° \\
- 1.00 \times 90° \\
\hline
+5.47 - 1.36 \times 90°
\end{array}
$$

SOLUTION:

$+5.47D - 1.36D \times 90°$

PROBLEM:

A lens of $-3.00 + 1.00 \times 180°$ is tilted pantoscopically $20°$. What is the effective power?

PROCEDURE:

Since the cylinder axis is $180°$, the total power of the cylinder is in the vertical meridian. By transposing the lens formula $-3.00 + 1.00 \times 180°$ to $-2.00 - 1.00 \times 90°$ it is seen that the power in the vertical meridian is $-2.00D$.

1.   Determine the power of the new sphere.

$$F_{n.s.} = F_{o.s.}(1 + \tfrac{1}{3}\sin^2 \Theta)$$

$$= -2.00(1 + \tfrac{1}{3}\sin^2 20°)$$

$$= -2.078D$$

2.   Determine the power of the induced cylinder.

$$F_{i.c.} = F_{o.s.}(\tan^2 \Theta)$$

$$= -2.00(\tan^2 20°)$$

$$= -0.264D$$

3. The induced power is $-2.078 - 0.264 \times 180°$, transposed it is $-2.342 + 0.264 \times 90°$.

4. Combine with cylinder of the transposed form in the original problem.

$$
\begin{array}{r}
-\ 1.00 \times 90° \\
\underline{-2.342 + 0.264 \times 90°} \\
-2.342 - 0.736 \times 90°
\end{array}
$$

PRACTICAL CONSIDERATIONS

The problems are given to demonstrate the effect of a pantoscopic angle. From a practical viewpoint, computations are usually not necessary when determining a prescription. The high correction is placed in a trial frame, which is adjusted at the spectacle plane. The practitioner then refines to give the best visual acuity before writing the final prescription.

WRAP-AROUND FRAME DESIGNS

Wrap-around, goggle-type frame designs result in a distortion similar to that of the pantoscopic tilt. However, the problem of distortion is more acute because these frames are designed with a wrap-around angle as high as 35°. The resultant longitudinal peripheral distortion can be intolerable to the patient.

The formulas demonstrating the power change in wrap-around eyewear are the same as those involved in the pantoscopic tilt except for the following change. Since the lenses are tilted about the vertical axis, the power in the horizontal meridian is affected; therefore, the induced cylinder is axis 90°.

PROBLEM:

The patient wears a prescription O.U. $+4.00 - 0.50 \times 90°$. If the correction is duplicated in a goggle-type sunframe that angles toward the face 15°, what is the resultant effective power?

PROCEDURE:

1. Transpose to determine the power at 180°.

    $$+3.50 + 0.50 \times 180°$$

2. Determine the power of the new sphere.

    $$F_{n.s.} = F_{o.s.}(1 + \tfrac{1}{3}\sin^2 \Theta)$$
    $$= +3.50(1 + \tfrac{1}{3}\sin^2 15°)$$
    $$= +3.577D$$

3. Determine the power of the induced cylinder.

    $$F_{i.c.} = F_{o.s.}(\tan^2 \Theta)$$
    $$= +3.50(\tan^2 15°)$$
    $$= +0.252D$$

4. Induced power $= +3.577 + 0.252 \times 90°$
    Transpose and combine with cylinder from step (1)

    $$
    \begin{array}{r}
    +3.829 - 0.252 \times 180° \\
    + 0.50 \times 180° \\
    \hline
    +3.829 + 0.248 \times 180°
    \end{array}
    $$

SOLUTION:

$+4.077 - 0.248 \times 90°$ (in original form)

PROBLEM:

A lens of $-5.00 + 1.00 \times 180°$ is duplicated in a wrap-around frame tilted 25° toward the temples. What is the resultant effective power?

PROCEDURE:

1.   Determine the power of the new sphere.

$$F_{n.s.} = F_{o.s.}(1 + \frac{1}{3}\sin^2 \Theta)$$
$$= -5.00(1 + \frac{1}{3}\sin^2 25°)$$
$$= -5.30D$$

2.   Determine the power of the induced cylinder.

$$F_{i.c.} = F_{o.s.}(\tan^2 \Theta)$$
$$= -5.00(\tan^2 25°)$$
$$= +1.085D$$

3.   Induced power $= -5.30 - 1.085 \times 90°$
4.   Transpose induced power to axis 180°.

$$-6.385 + 1.085 \times 180°$$

5.   Combine with original cylinder.

$$
\begin{array}{r}
-6.385 + 1.085 \times 180° \\
+ 1.00 \times 180° \\
\hline
-6.385 + 2.085 \times 180°
\end{array}
$$

SOLUTION:

$-6.385 + 2.085 \times 180°$

The above example clearly shows that the prescription change caused by angling of a lens can be disturbing to the patient.

Sensitivity to the wrap-around angle when low-power lenses are involved varies with the individual. Some patients find almost any horizontal distortion intolerable, particularly when operating a motor vehicle; others will ignore the aberration if the amount is not too great. Fortunately, the problem has been lessened with the current availability of great numbers of chic sunframes that are not curved toward the temples.

Chapter 15

LENS DESIGNS AND CONTEMPORARY EYE FRAMES

INTRODUCTION

The wide variety of materials used in the manufacture of contemporary eyewear has made possible the greatest choice of frame fashions in history. Almost every basic design of every era has been expanded to meet modern styling needs ranging from the conventional to the avant-garde. For decades the majority of frames were made of plastic or metal. While this is still true, there are other materials and designs that are slowly overtaking the field with titanium being especially popular. Sometimes certain types of lenses offer definite advantages when used in conjunction with specific frame types. This chapter includes a discussion of contemporary stylings with recommendations about lenses providing the best service to the patient.

PLASTIC FRAMES

Frames fashioned of zylonite (cellulose acetate) and usually referred to as *zyl* are among the most popular contemporary designs. They are often the choice of famous designers because they lend themselves admirably to the beauty of haute couture.

Zylonite/zyl was and still is the most used material for plastic frames. It can be produced inexpensively in an almost unlimited variety of colors and textures. In addition, it is easy to work with and easy to adjust on the patient's face. Because of its flexibility all lens designs can be accommodated by zylonite/zyl. However, there are other frames, discussed later, that may prove more serviceable. Continued contact with cosmetics and perspiration can discolor zylonite. Zylonite frames also tend to fade when subjected over a period of time to sun and heat. It is probably best to seriously consider recommending a newer type of frame material.

Optyl, introduced in Europe during the late 1960s, was marketed extensively in the United States for several decades. In many ways it is a remarkable plastic material. Optyl retains its beauty almost indefinitely; it is not affected by exposure to the elements, such as sun and wind. Secretions of the skin—perspiration/oil—do not change the appearance of Optyl; neither does hair spray. Therefore, the grayish films that often form on zylonite frames, particularly along the temples, are absent. Unlike some other frame materials, Opytl is hypoallergenic; there has not been a single case on record of a skin rash resulting from optyl mountings. Optyl is comfortable to wear, weighing about one-third less than a comparable zylonite frame. Once adjusted, Optyl keeps its alignment indefinitely unless reheated, whereby it goes back to its original factory shape (it has complete memory). CR 39 plastic lenses have less bitoric effect when used with Optyl than with other frame materials that surround the lenses. In every tested sampling, the eyewear conforms to ANSI standards for ophthalmic prescriptions. It is not more widely used because some manufacturers have exclusive rights to the material.

Although the current fashion look in eyewear spotlights the small designs, there are patients who prefer larger mountings, particularly for sunwear. Plastic frames with a rigid-pad bridge construction, particularly the Optyl designs, when coupled with CR 39 or polycarbonate lenses offer the ultimate in comfort. Such frames may work with some glass lenses to provide comfortable eyewear, although glass sometimes presents weight problems, particularly with high-index designs and photochromic lenses.

Plastic frames result in the best cosmetic look for high minus and prism corrections because the rims cover much of the edges. When the lenses are tinted a hue in the same color family as the primary shade of the frame to eliminate the sharp line of demarcation between lenses and mounting, the cosmetic effect is the best possible.

Note: Occasionally, on a limited basis, other plastics besides zylonite and Optyl are introduced into the fashion frame field. It is always necessary to check with the manufacturer for specifics. For example, cellulose propionate requires less heat for adjusting than zylonite because overheating can damage the frame. The designs have no memory. If stretched they will not return to original size or shape, so the mounting is ruined.

METAL AND GOLD-FILLED MOUNTINGS (WIRES)

In the 1940s through the middle 1950s, frames featuring metal rims surrounding the lenses were dispensed almost exclusively to industrial workers whose occupations made durability a prime concern. In the late 1950s and early 1960s these industrial frames were replaced largely by plastic designs because most workers during that period preferred their cosmetic appeal. In addition, since industrial-thickness glass lenses were almost always prescribed, plastic frames resulted in more comfortable eyewear. Metal mountings had adjustable-pad bridge designs, and these small contact areas carrying most of the weight of the glasses often left sore marks on the nose.

A dramatic reappearance of these metal frames took place about the middle to late 1960s. Spurred by the hippie movement, many teenagers and young college students sought these obsolete styles in shops specializing in "elegant junk," bringing them into professional offices for lens prescriptions. Optical manufacturers, recognizing marketing potential, added a touch of fashion to the basic designs and introduced narrow "granny" wires. The popularity of metal frames is still here, with current designs featuring primarily a narrow look, but some having a deep vertical dimension. In offices concerned with fashion, metal frames often appear to be overwhelmingly the choice of patients, far surpassing the plastic designs.

Some metal mounting designs are constructed with a plastic bridge, but the vast majority have an adjustable-pad bridge construction. When glass lenses are mounted into the latter, patients frequently complain of nasal pressure as well as unsightly red marks on the nose. Sometimes the complaints are severe, especially if the lenses are oversize, thicker than conventional (i.e., photochromics or high-power corrections) or if the patient has undergone rhinoplasty (nose surgery). Plastic lenses, particularly polycarbonates, are the most satisfactory choice for wire frames. In the past, high minus or prism corrections were not cosmetically suitable for wirelike frames because the edges are almost completely exposed. The newer plastic, high index, aspheric lenses, however, can be very attractive in these mountings.

The use of a light tint can often enhance the fashion value of eyewear utilizing metal mountings. The hues that look best while keeping the visible spectrum relatively intact are pale pinks, soft grays, and very light tans. Some practitioners may order polished lens edges for cosmetic value, but there are patients who do not like that look.

It is sometimes tempting to recommend high-index glass lenses for the high myope who insists on a wire mounting. This is rarely a satisfactory procedure. Although the lenses are relatively thin, they are comparatively heavy. This is especially annoying if the mounting is a large-eye fashion and has an adjustable-pad bridge construction. (The use of the brittle flint glass, Thinlite, in single-vision and one-piece multifocal lenses was eliminated with the FDA ruling regarding impact-resistant lenses. The newer high-index glass, distributed under various trade names, can be chemically tempered.) However, polycarbonate lenses or other high-index plastic lenses are the best choice. They have excellent cosmetic value and can be tinted many beautiful shades.

COMBINATION AND COMBINATION-TYPE MOUNTINGS

An amazing development was the emerging of combination and combination-type frames into the world of fashion eyewear. The former are "factory worker" mountings issued since the 1940s; the latter have been primarily an "older person" mounting, especially for the low-vision patient. Both designs are characterized by metal rims (called a *chassis*) circling the lenses. Combination mountings are topped by wide zylonite bars and usually have zylonite temples. Combination-type frames feature aluminum tops/temples. Both are "small" eye fashions, almost always with 52mm as the largest available eye size. The bridges have an adjustable pad construction.

In 1986 (and continuing to this day), these frames began appearing on the faces of theatrical personalities, particularly "rock stars" who favored the designs. Because of the adjustable pad construction, it is always best to use plastic lenses, especially since the lenses are almost always tinted an unusual color that is easily achieved on plastic.

TITANIUM FRAMES

The most dramatic recent change in the eyewear field is the use of titanium for fashion frames. Titanium not only produces beautiful modern designs but also is a remarkable material. It is twice as strong as stainless steel yet is about 45% lighter, making it very comfortable on the face. There is also a health benefit for some patients. Nickel, a common element in some metal frames, causes allergic reactions in many patients. The resultant skin rash is not only unsightly but also painful. Titanium frames are hypoallergenic and should be seriously considered if the patient gives a history of dermatitis. Fortunately, there are also great styling possibilities with these corrosion-resistant frames. Titanium frames take color beautifully and therefore are available in the newest shades that keep up with fashion trends.

RIMLESS AND SEMI-RIMLESS DESIGNS

In the 1930s and 1940s the most popular frames were rimless-type mountings. Lens edges were completely exposed. Most featured a bar (sometimes called an *arm*) that curved upward from the bridge to follow along and behind the upper edges of the lens. Others were what manufacturers call a *complete rimless*. The bar was absent and the lenses attached to the mounting at four points, two nasal and two temporal. In the 1950s, they were replaced by plastic frames and it became rare to see patients wearing rimless designs. In the 1960s, the hippie movement brought rimless along with wire mountings back into fashion. The popularity of these frames has continued to this day, and the passing decades have spotlighted consistently updated, elegant versions.

Plastic lenses serve particularly well in rimless designs. In fact, some laboratories will not fill prescriptions asking for drilled glass lenses, because the lenses readily break at the points of attachment. It is not unusual for patients in the entertainment field to request unusual shapes (resembling hearts, flowers, etc.), and CR 39 plastic can be hand-formed easily to almost any desired pattern.

When high-minus lenses or prism corrections are involved, the appearance of the exposed thick edges can present a problem. If cosmetic value is critical, it may be best to recommend a frame design that covers the bevels, although controlling the lens size is a possible answer. As a guide, a −4.00D CR 39 hard-resin lens having a 54mm horizontal box measurement will be about 6mm thick on the temporal edges. Fortunately, the most requested 46mm eye and 48mm eye in rimless designs, which appear to be the current fashion choice, limit the problem. The newer high-index plastic lenses should be seriously considered and often are suitable for these designs.

Rimless designs can also be "nylon-suspension" frames. These feature a clear nylon thread that circles the lenses. Breakage is almost impossible because the lenses are not drilled, and glass designs, such as photochromics, can be used if desired. Polycarbonate lenses are an excellent recommendation. There may be problems, however, with some bevels, such as those on laminated lenses. If in doubt, it is best to query the laboratory.

While at one time, lenses in a rimless frame were fashion tinted, most patients now ask for clear lenses. If desired, some of the color effects, such as gradient tints and two tones in juxtaposition, easily achieved with CR 39 lenses, can be stunning on deep-shaped patterns. The range in tint possibilities for polycarbonates has greatly expanded, and most colors are now available.

Complete rimless mountings are almost always the choice of patients desiring jeweling on a lens since the absence of rims focuses attention on the design. The lenses must be CR 39. The jewels should be small and placed on the lower temporal corner of one lens so as not to interfere with vision. Tinted lenses can serve as the fashion background. In the 1970s this effect was extremely popular, particularly the personalized jeweled initials, but the late 1980s showed a slowdown. However, by the year 2000, jeweling on lenses was spotlighted in fashion magazines, worn by celebrities, and again requested by some patients.

ALUMINUM FRAMES

Aluminum frames are rarely dispensed today but may return as high fashion. The gold- and silver-appearing designs look like elegant jewelry. Those featuring high fashion colors lend themselves to a contemporary look. Half-eye aluminum mountings are especially striking in these gorgeous shades. Aluminum is a rigid metal, and plastic lenses are best in most of these designs. However, some wearers of the half-eyes may prefer glass lenses because of the frequent "off-and-on" process. While a full-size aluminum frame is not necessarily heavier than a plastic design, it is seldom as comfortable. This probably results from the feeling of metal against the skin. The patient is best served when polycarbonate lenses are recommended in these full-size fashions.

NYLON FRAMES

The allure of nylon frames is that they are almost indestructible, and while they tend to look like zyl, they are much lighter. However, a number of considerations may limit their use. Although the frame colors have been drastically improved, they rarely meet the beauty possibilities of zylonite plastic, the material they most resemble visually. Nylon is difficult to adjust with conventional frame-heating devices. (Manufacturers recommend using hot water.) In very cold weather nylon may become brittle and crack. The solution, according to manufacturers, is immersing the eyewear in water overnight several times a week so that dehydration does not take place. Obviously, this is not always convenient.

Some of the newer nylon frames are created from blended nylon families (polyamides, co-polyamides, and gliamides). These virtually eliminate the dryness issue and should be used if at all possible. They also allow for greater variation in achieving attractive colors.

A special nylon sport frame has a rubberized nose/bridge area and riding-bow temples that, when held on the head with an athletic strap hooked through the temples, proves highly efficient for the patient engaged in contact sports. For safety's sake, plastic lenses should be mounted in this design. While nylon clamps down on hard-resin prescription lenses creating a relatively high bitoric effect, the eyewear, limited to sporting activities, is rarely worn long enough to give rise to aesthenopia.

A number of manufacturers are making available nylon frames with plano polycarbonate lenses for use as active-wear fashions. These are the safest form of eyewear available and make the best use of nylon frames.

Note: In all testing of CR 39 prescription lenses mounted into the older nylon frames, the bitoric effect was too high to meet the standards set by ANSI.

Nylon is sometimes combined with rubber for sports eyewear. These frames are soft and comfortable but do not allow for frame adjustments. They must be a perfect fit during the frame selection process.

HALF-EYE FRAMES

Half-eye frames are used as "reading prescription" eyewear. Designed to be small—usually a 46mm, 48mm, or 50mm eyesize—they are worn low on the nose, enabling the patient to look over them for distant viewing. Contemporary half-eyes are available in aluminum, plastic, nylon, metal (wire), and rimless styles. Glass may be the lens of choice because half-eyes are often subjected to the taking-off/putting-on process, making a highly scratch-resistant lens the most practical. Weight should not present a problem since the frame is small and the correction is rarely greater than +2.50D.

When the half-eye frame is fashioned of aluminum or metal or is a drilled rimless mounting, plastic lenses should be considered because edge chipping is a consideration. Coatings that make the front surface of CR 39 as scratch resistant as glass are easily available. Quality polycarbonate lenses have factory-placed coatings that make them very practical and can be an excellent recommendation.

Half-eye eyewear utilizing spherical corrections, ranging from +1.00D to +2.50D can be purchased over-the-counter in most drug stores. More elegant designs are often sold in fashionable boutiques and at cosmetic counters in department stores. The lenses may not meet ophthalmic standards but are satisfactory for short-term reading tasks. When half-eyes are used for prolonged reading, the patient should be encouraged to order proper prescription lenses to insure comfort.

LORGNETTES

Lorgnettes are designed to be held before the eyes when a presbyope needs momentary clear vision. They are usually fashioned of plastic or gold-filled metal. When not in use, most fold at the bridge, with the lenses slipping into a hollow handle. They are used primarily by women who display them as styled accessories, as when reading a dinner menu, glancing at a theater program, etc.

Lenses mounted into a lorgnette frame must be ground with flat base curves if they are to fit properly into the handle. Glass is the only suitable choice because it is difficult, if not impossible, to order the desired curvature in plastic lenses.

It may be best to recommend lorgnette frames with lenses already mounted into them. A few optical concerns stock them with glass lenses of powers +1.50D spheres, +2.00D spheres, and +2.50D spheres. It is rarely necessary to order the patient's exact near correction because the eyewear is used only minutes at a time. Practically speaking, it is unusual for a woman to order lorgnettes from a practitioner. They are purchased as elegant fashion accessories from boutiques or upscale department stores.

FRAME CONSIDERATIONS IN MULTIFOCAL PRESCRIBING

It is always a concern when frame fashions concentrate on a narrow-appearing design (difference of 10mm or greater between the horizontal A and vertical B measurements) because there is difficulty in giving the multifocal patient a suitable near area. With such frames, clinical experience reveals that wider segments should be ordered for compensation. If a flat-top segment is 13mm high, the horizontal bifocal measurement should be at least 28mm; if the trifocal height is 19mm, a straight-top 7 × 28mm is the best for general wear.

Fortunately, contemporary eyeframes spotlight so many designs that deep lens shapes allowing for a higher segment are easily available. It is not unusual to order general-wear bifocals 19mm, 20mm, and 21mm high (the segment line positioned just below or at the lower lid for easy neck and head posturing). The intermediate segment in a trifocal is customarily 7mm in depth, so an overall height of 22mm (usually the intermediate line is about 1mm below the lower pupil margin in normal indoor illumination) allows for a comfortable 15mm-high near segment.

When prescribing seamless (blended) bifocals, it is important to use a frame with a deep vertical dimension. The blur circle that separates the distance from the near correction is easier to ignore when the ordered segment height is at least 20mm.

Although most progressive addition lenses need a frame allowing a minimum of 22mm from the pupil center to the lower lens edge, a mounting providing a longer measurement gives the patient a larger near field.

In the late 1990s, progressive addition lenses that can be worn with a shorter vertical frame dimension were made available. Discussion of measurements for individual progressive addition lenses is found in Chapter 5, "Prescribing 'Invisible' Multifocals."

Interestingly, patients who desire progressive addition lenses for their cosmetic value (absence of segment dividing lines) are also highly concerned with the fashion value of the frame. When narrow-shaped frames are used, it is always best to recommend a separate pair with the accurate full prescription for prolonged near work.

All occupational multifocals require frames with a deep vertical dimension allowing for the necessary "high segment" positioning. Fortunately, such designs are widely available, often with adjustable pads that allow the lenses to be set precisely for better patient satisfaction.

CONCLUSION

It is obvious to everyone in the eyecare field that popular frame designs are always associated with name designer (e.g., Calvin Klein) or a famous personality (e.g., Sophia Loren, Gloria Vanderbilt). This trend, which started a number of decades ago, will undoubtedly continue indefinitely.

Patients enjoy these designs always fashioned of a popular frame material. They add class to eyewear, which in the past was considered a necessary prosthetic. The designer's touch/famed person connection is a great asset to the eyecare field, especially when combined with the best cosmetically appearing lens designs.

Chapter 16

FRAME ADJUSTMENTS— ENSURING INTEGRITY OF THE LENS OPTICS

INTRODUCTION

To insure that the prescribed lenses deliver maximum efficiency, proper adjustment of the eyewear is critical. The frame must angle correctly on the face for the optics to perform as intended. There are also valuable benefits to proper alignment. The beauty of the eyewear, an integral factor in today's fashion frames, is enhanced as frames appearing crooked on the face look awkward and unappealing. Comfort is also involved. If the nose pads are not positioned properly, for example, the eyewear can feel "annoying." The optics of the lenses can be compromised if the frame angles incorrectly toward the patient's temples.

In this book titled *Practical Aspects of Ophthalmic Optics*, therefore, a most practical aspect is the inclusion of a chapter involving frame alignments and adjustments.

Specifically designed optical tools for frame alignment/adjustment are a necessity. Tool kits are widely available from optical distributors. Most of the kits have a minimum of ten different pliers each designed for a specific use. Instructions/explanation accompany each tool. The name of the tool also gives a clue as to its use (e.g., angling pliers). Eyecare professionals often add their own favorites to these basics. These can be purchased separately.

ALIGNMENT PROCEDURES

Eyewear should always be aligned before being adjusted on the face. This greatly simplifies angling for facial contours to insure a good fit. Optical laboratories should send the eyewear correctly aligned, but since this does not always happen, the following steps *done in the order given* insure that alignment of one part of the frame is compatible to the alignment of another.

ALIGNMENT OF METAL MOUNTINGS

(Some specific characteristics of certain metals are discussed later in this chapter.)

1. If the metal mounting (sometimes called wire mounting) shows convexity, concavity, and/or a propeller effect, adjust at the bridge *with the fingers* until a straight edge (usually the optical ruler is used) placed horizontally on the inside surface touches the nasal and temporal extremities of the eyewear.

    Note: Some popular sunwear designs show concavity with respect to perfect alignment. This angle is created for a fashion look and is only appropriate with plano lenses. If prescription lenses are involved, the angle causes peripheral distortion and, in higher prescriptions, seriously affects the patient's vision (see Chapter 14 "Prescription Changes Induced by Lens Tilt").

2. The temple spread should be equal on both sides. It can be increased or decreased by bending the endpieces with the proper designated tool. Do not bend

the temple itself unless absolutely necessary because this can result in an unsightly look. While the actual angle is determined when the eyewear is fit on the face, it is usually best to start with the temples perpendicular to the frame front.

3. The pantoscopic angle (the lower portion of the frame angled toward the cheeks) is usually best at a 5° bend. Holding the endpiece with the proper pliers, bend the temple up or down with the fingers until the desired effect is achieved. When placed on a flat surface, the temples and tops of the lenses should touch simultaneously.

4. Metal mountings almost always have adjustable pads. When the pads are viewed from the ocular side of the eyewear, the lower edges should diverge about 45° with the face of the pad also angled by about 45° and fully visible. This angle will follow the nose bridges of most patients, although flat bridges or asymmetric noses (usually the result of injuries) will require additional alignment.

ALIGNMENT OF RIMLESS MOUNTINGS

There are two basic kinds of rimless mountings. The most popular, known as the complete rimless, features a four-point attachment of the lenses. Each lens is attached at two places, nasally at the nose bridge and temporally at the endpieces. Extreme caution is needed when aligning these mountings because the lenses can "snap" at the point of attachment even when plastic lenses are involved.

Other rimless designs feature a bar (sometimes called an *arm*) that follows along and usually behind the top of the lenses. (Some designers, however, place a widened, decorated bar in front of the lenses for a fashion look.) There are usually only two points of attachment, one on each lens at the nasal bridge area. Both the four-point attachment and the two point attachment mountings are aligned in the same manner.

1. If the eyewear shows concavity, convexity, or a propeller effect, bend at the bridge with the fingers until a straight edge (usually a short, rigid optical ruler) placed horizontally on the inside surface touches the nasal and temporal extremities.

2. The narrow bar (or arm) in a conventional design should curve along and behind the upper portion of the lenses clearing by about 1mm. If this curvature is not done properly at the laboratory, it is probably best to return the eyewear for correct bar placement. The lenses need to be remounted by an expert technician. If the decorated (and sometimes jeweled) bar is in front of the lenses, alignment must always be done by an expert.

3. The temples should angle evenly from the front of the mounting. While the actual angle is determined by the shape of the patient's head, it is best to start with the temples perpendicular to the front. Bend at the end-pieces for this alignment using the pliers designed for this purpose.

4. Place the eyewear on a flat surface. The temples and the top of the lenses should touch the surface simultaneously. Bend at the endpieces to make the proper alignment.

5. Rimless mountings almost always have an adjustable-pad bridge construction. When the eyewear is viewed from the ocular side, the lower edges of the pads should diverge about 45° with the face of the pad fully visible (angled about 45°). Place the pads in this position by bending the pad arms. These angles are a good starting point for contouring to the patient's nose.

ALIGNMENT OF PLASTIC FRAMES

1. The front of the frame should not show concavity, convexity, or a propeller effect. If alignment is necessary, form a "hill" with the hot salt in the "salt pan" designed for use in adjustment of plastic frames. Heat only the bridge, being careful not to place the rims in the hot salt (the lenses may fall out) and bend with the fingers to the proper alignment.

2. Temples should be perpendicular to the front. If the frame features a hidden-hinge temple that needs to be angled in, heat the endpiece and bend with the fingers. If the hinge is exposed, grasp it with pliers designed for this purpose. If the temple spread needs to be increased, use a "rough" optical file and file in

one direction only. A sawing motion can ruin the look of the plastic. Do this slowly and gradually so that the angle spread does not become too great. The final angle position will be made on the patient's face during the adjustment procedure.

3.   The pantoscopic angle with the lower edges of the eyewear toward the cheeks should be about 5°. For a hidden-hinge construction, increase or decrease the angle by bending *unheated* temples up or down with the fingers. *Do not heat endpieces or temples.* This can loosen the hinges and make the frame impossible to repair. The eyewear will then wobble on the patient's face and never stay in proper adjustment. If the hinge is exposed, grasp the endpiece with the pliers and bend the temples up or down with the fingers. Again, *do not heat.*

4.   There tends to be a fashion return to plastic frames that have jewels imbedded directly into the plastic. Before placing the jeweled area in the salt pan, check with the manufacturer to see if a clear plastic coating protects the stones. It is best never to place a jeweled frame in hot salt if it does not have this coating because the stones may fall out. If the manufacturer is unknown (the patient may have purchased the frame in a foreign country), an alignment/adjusting procedure that involves any of the jeweled portion should not be tried. Some manufacturers send extra "jewels" when the frame is ordered, but these are difficult to place properly if the original jeweling is "disturbed."

SPECIAL NOTE REGARDING OPTYL PLASTIC FRAMES

Optyl frames will be identified as such inside the temples. These frames must be heated to a rubbery consistency before bending. If bending is forced, the plastic will break. Optyl also has the property of "complete memory" meaning that reheating nullifies the original adjustment, and the plastic reverts to its factory shape. It takes skill to make the correct adjustment with each try. A heated Optyl frame should never be cooled by placing in cold water (this can be done with zylonite plastic frames) because the Optyl is likely to break. Air cooling is an absolute necessity.

ALIGNMENT OF ALUMINUM FRAMES

At one time, almost all high-fashion frames were constructed of aluminum. While few of those designs are still manufactured, there is a current "craze" in fashion that reverts back to the 1950s and 1960s, when these expensive fashions were widely worn. Boutiques selling these frames (along with the jewelry of those years) are flourishing, particularly in the Los Angeles/Beverly Hills and New York areas.

1. If an aluminum frame is seriously out of alignment, it is almost impossible to achieve a proper fit. It is best to advise the patient of the problem and not attempt alignment. If only minor changes are necessary, all adjustments must be made with the fingers or rubber-coated pliers so as not to mar the aluminum.

2. The front is not likely to show convexity or concavity or have a propeller effect unless it is seriously damaged. If it does, bend the bridge *very slowly* so the aluminum does not crackle. If this alignment is not almost perfect, it is best not to use the frame at all, because only slight pressure can be applied.

3. If the temples need to be angled out, do not file the temple butt because that will remove the color. Bend *slowly* at the endpieces with the fingers remembering that the angle placed at the factory level can be altered only slightly.

4. The pantoscopic angle is changed by bending at the endpieces with the fingers. However, only a slight change is possible. Usually the angle placed at the factory level needs to fit the patient properly, and this is determined during the frame selection process.

TITANIUM FRAMES

More and more manufacturers are making available high-fashion titanium frames. Sometimes the material is mixed with nickel alloy, but the patient may be allergic to nickel. The face can swell, the skin break out in a rash. (This is the reason manufacturers of quality jewelry no longer mix gold with nickel but find other alloys for their designs.) Nickel is the most common culprit of contact allergies. It is estimated that 10% to 15% of the population is sensitive to it. It is always best to recommend titanium frames that do not have a nickel alloy.

Titanium frames are ultralight, so they are welcomed by patients with sensitive nose bridges (especially if they have had rhinoplasty—the cosmetic procedure to alter nose shape/size). Older patients also enjoy the comfort these frames offer. Other important advantages are that they tend to retain their beauty and need little if any adjustment. If a titanium frame accidentally bends, it will return to its original shape, so in the selection process, it should be a perfect fit.

STAINLESS STEEL FRAMES

This material is gaining great popularity in frame design. It combines flexibility with durability and can be made extremely thin in keeping with contemporary fashion trends. The metal has a springy effect, which tends to make the temples rest easily on the face. Stainless steel frames are easy to align for a comfortable fit.

INDUSTRIAL AND SPORT FRAMES

These frame designs must be received in perfect alignment from the manufacturer. Trying to change alignment is almost impossible. Most in this category are frames for industrial (safety) use and sport frames. Fortunately, these often are made of a "give" material that will conform to a degree to the wearer's face.

These frames are almost always released with safety plano lenses. The practitioner should hesitate about trying to replace these lenses with a prescription.

EYEWEAR ADJUSTMENT ON THE PATIENT'S FACE

When a frame alignment is done properly, adjustments on the face to make the eyewear fit comfortably and have aesthetic value should be relatively simple. The adjustment procedure is the same for all frame designs. *All steps must be done in the following order:*

1. Nose pads are adjusted first.

    a. The proper fit of a rigid-pad frame is usually determined when the patient selects the frame. Sometimes, however, the pad angle can be slightly modified. Heat the pad in a big spoon filled with hot salt and *slowly* bend to the desired position. (If the pad breaks off, it is almost always necessary to order a new frame.)

    b. Adjustable pads should be placed just short of the inner canthi. To insure comfort, *the entire face of the pad* should touch the nose area. Angling the lower portion about 45° is best for most patients. Looking at the patient, no part of the pad face should be visible. Lift the eyewear slightly off the nose and adjust the pads to clear the inner canthi by about 1mm. If when the frame is moved back and forth, the pads still touch the nose, the eyewear will not be comfortable for patients with sensitive nose bridges. In some cases soft, cushiony pad covers that are available in suitable sizes may be necessary.

2. The eyewear should appear straight on the face (except for the patient with a hyper eye where a modification may be necessary). The cheeks should be used as a guideline (not the eyebrows). A lens is lowered by *raising* the temple on the corresponding side or *lowering* the temple on the opposite side. For aesthetic value, bend at the endpiece, not the temple itself.

3. Each lens should be the same distance away from the face. To bring the right lens closer, turn the left temple *in* or the right temple *out* by bending at the endpieces. Reverse the process if the left lens needs to be closer.

4. The temples should rest gently on the side of the head neither indenting the flesh or be bowed out in a clumsy manner. Except for the straight-back design, they should be contoured carefully behind the ears for a comfortable fit.

    a. Skull temples are used on most frames. There is a characteristic bend meant for the top of the ear. If the temples are too short, this bend comes before the ear and is unsightly. When the patient selects a frame, this factor should be taken into consideration. (Unfortunately, this is not always the case as noted by the number of politicians, guests, etc., on television programs who have not been fit properly.)

b. Straight back temples (also known as library or spatula temples). There is little adjustment necessary for this design. Since this temple is meant for easy "on-off" it needs only slight contouring behind the ears. Straight-back temples are usually found on sunwear fashions and eyewear used for reading. They tend to go out of adjustment easily, and this factor should be considered when recommending a frame using this design.

c. Comfort cable temples (also known as Relaxo temples). These designs feature coiled metal that curves around the ears. They are almost always used on frames that need extra security to stay on the face (e.g., sports and activewear designs). The metal should be shaped with the fingers to contour behind the ears. Angle the ends up slightly (using pliers) so they do not to dig into the patient's flesh. Eyecare professionals often slip a cover over the metal that goes behind the ears to make the temples more comfortable.

d. Riding bow temples. These are used almost exclusively on children's zylonite frames. They are made of a thin plastic and have a characteristic wire core. When the temples are new, contouring behind the child's ears can be done without heating, but as the frame ages, the plastic becomes brittle. Breakage can occur if the temples are not heated for a necessary adjustment. These designs rarely last longer than a year before the plastic cracks, but by that time, the child will have outgrown the frame.

e. Metal temples with ends coated in plastic. These temples are almost always a skull design. Warming the ends may be necessary, but if overheated the metal core will burn the plastic. Extreme caution is necessary when adjusting these designs.

5.   For optical and cosmetic reasons, eyewear should angle pantoscopically on the face. If the lower edges need to be closer to the cheeks, bend the temples down *evenly* making sure that the lower edges of the eyewear do not touch the face. If this occurs, angle *both* temples up to correct the problem.

6.   When bifocals, trifocals, or any multifocal is involved, it is critical that the eyewear be adjusted so that the segments for each eye are reached simultaneously when the patient reaches these areas.

Note: If the eyewear causes any kind of a contact allergy (mild itching, redness, sometimes even severe infection), the patient is allergic to the frame. While this can occur with any material, including plastics, the most likely culprit is nickel added to other metal material in the manufacturing process. The frame should be replaced immediately.

CONCLUSION

With all frame fashions, the fit is critical to insuring the optics of the eyewear. The optics and thus the lens effectivity changes when the frame angles incorrectly on the face. Obviously, the attractiveness of the fashion is also compromised. For these reasons, the patient should return at about 6-month intervals for realignment because the putting-on, taking-off process can, and often does, alter fit.

It needs also to be noted here that other frame materials are likely to be released in the future. It is critical to study the literature accompanying each design to understand the adjustable properties.

INDEX

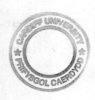

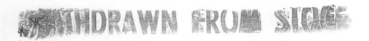